Belli Beautiful

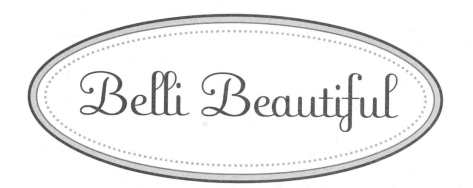

Belli Beautiful

The Essential Guide to the Safest Health and Beauty Products for Pregnancy, Mom, and Baby

Annette Rubin and Melissa Schweiger

Foreword by Jason Rubin, MD

Da Capo
LIFE
LONG
A Member of the Perseus Books Group

Design by Brent Wilcox

Library of Congress Cataloging-in-Publication Data
Rubin, Annette.
    Belli beautiful : the essential guide to safe and healthy personal care products for pregnancy, mom, and baby / Annette Rubin and Melissa Schweiger ; foreword by Jason Rubin.
        p.   cm.
    Includes bibliographical references and index.
    ISBN 978-0-7382-1491-7 (paperback)—ISBN 978-0-7382-1580-8 (e-book)
    1. Pregnancy—Popular works.   2. Skin—Care and hygiene—Popular works.   3. Self-care, Health—Popular works.   I. Schweiger, Melissa.   II. Title.
    RG525.R83 2012
    649'.10242—dc23

                                                                            2011050795

First Da Capo Press edition 2012

Published by Da Capo Press
A Member of the Perseus Books Group
www.dacapopress.com

Da Capo Press books are available at special discounts for bulk purchases in the U.S. by corporations, institutions, and other organizations. For more information, please contact the Special Markets Department at the Perseus Books Group, 2300 Chestnut Street, Suite 200, Philadelphia, PA 19103, or call (800) 810-4145, ext. 5000, or e-mail special.markets@perseusbooks.com.

This book is dedicated to the strongest
and most beautiful women we know—moms!

Contents

Foreword

by Jason Rubin, MD

About twelve years ago, when my wife Annette became pregnant with our first son, she asked me about the safety of different topical ingredients while expecting. She was using about ten skin care and twelve cosmetic products a day, each with over a dozen different ingredients, and she wanted to know which of those chemicals were okay and which she should try to avoid. My first thought was that the skin care companies were probably being very cautious with their ingredient choices. Physicians have known for decades that chemicals in creams and lotions can pass through the skin and enter the bloodstream. Surely the skin care industry wouldn't ignore the risks of topical absorption and the possible effects on the growing baby during pregnancy.

Out of curiosity, I started calling around to different companies and asking questions. Are your ingredients safe for pregnancy? Are they absorbed through the skin? How do you know for sure? I was shocked by the answers. All of the companies I spoke with said that their products were safe during pregnancy because they weren't absorbed, but they couldn't point to any research that backed up this claim. Nobody was screening the ingredients for links to birth defects or miscarriages. The experience had me wondering: what does "safe" really mean? In a world where our medical knowledge is constantly evolving, product safety is a moving target. Ingredients that we think are perfectly harmless today could be shown in research tomorrow to cause cancer, birth defects, or Alzheimer's disease. Or what about a medication that causes a serious side effect in 0.001 percent of the population? Most of us would consider this drug harmless—but not the handful of people who end up in the hospital after using it. It's enough to make you wonder: can we really say that anything is completely safe?

They say that medicine is an art as well as a science. That's definitely true. Physicians use research studies to learn more about the science behind the human body, but our understanding of its complex systems will never be complete. And that's where the art comes in—our job is to balance the many gaps in our knowledge with a patient's need for safe, sound advice.

We learn so much during medical school, but three pieces of wisdom have always stuck out in my mind. First, do no harm. Second, all bleeding stops—eventually. (Surgeons have a very strange sense of humor.) And third: when in doubt, always err on the side of caution.

I use each of these rules in my medical practice each day. The easiest visits are the ones where it's perfectly obvious what the problem is and which treatment is needed: fractures need splinting, lacerations need suturing, and heart attacks need quick medications and a rapid transfer to the cath lab. It's the other visits that keep me from sleeping at night—the diagnostic dilemmas for which there are dozens of possible explanations but no certainty about which one is right, even with all the expensive labs, X-rays, and other imaging studies.

When I'm seeing adult patients, I'm able to explain all the risks and benefits of each choice so the patient can make an informed decision. With children, however, the rules change. Children can't explain their symptoms very well, so I have to wonder there may be more going on. I'm even more cautious with infants and newborns—their little bodies are so fragile. Adults can accept a certain amount of risk in their lives, but we try not to take any chances when it comes to babies. I'll send an adult home with an unexplained fever and give him a few tablets of Tylenol, but I'll admit a two-month-old baby to the local children's hospital for the exact same thing. It just makes sense to be more careful with little ones, and that's *especially* true for the developing fetus during pregnancy. Their bodies are so tiny that even a small chemical exposure could be hazardous.

The more Annette and I thought about it, the more we realized that the world needs a higher safety standard for skin care products during pregnancy—one that errs on the side of caution. That was the moment when my wife and I realized that, as a beauty industry professional and a physician, we could make a real difference in people's lives. We could formulate a medically responsible line of skin care products for new moms and their babies. And that's when our company, Belli, was born.

Research moves slowly. There are so many chemicals to study, and most of the research dollars go to new medications. There's little push to study the safety of skin care ingredients that have been around for a while. When a research study does show that a cosmetic ingredient causes a birth defect, doctors often don't know what to do because most such experiments are done on animals—we can't say for sure that the same thing would happen in humans. At Belli, rather than wait for a topical ingredient to be proven harmful beyond doubt, we thought a more cautious approach would be for pregnant women to start avoiding questionable ingredients much sooner, when the first link to a birth defect or miscarriage has appeared in a published medical study, involving animals or humans, at any dose, and through any method of absorption. And thus Belli's *teratology screening* process was born.

Annette and I love what we created together at Belli, and we get really excited whenever we start working on a new product. There are always newer, more effective ingredients around the corner and new safety research that's yet to be uncovered! I keep track of all the latest medical research, and I update our formulations to stay ahead of the curve. But even so, every once in a while I'm asked a question that makes me think twice about a certain ingredient choice. I think that's great! Neither our products nor our information will ever be perfect, but that's part of the art of medicine too—caring enough to try.

I have learned so much about skin care safety over the last decade, especially as it relates to expecting moms and babies. Since there could never be enough space on the side of a cosmetic box to share all of this vital information, Annette, Melissa, and I are thrilled to be able to offer it in this book. With Melissa's passion for writing about beauty and our passion for understanding the safety of health and beauty products, we knew that the partnership was right. We hope this book will empower you to make smart choices each time you shop for skin care products. Whether it's our brand or another that we recommend, we want every woman to feel beautiful throughout pregnancy—and also to enjoy peace of mind.

Introduction

We are unabashed beauty fanatics. We're both skin care geeks who actually look forward to washing our faces at night. We love discovering the latest and greatest products on the market, and we have the careers to prove it: for decades, we've each been working in the beauty industry, learning about it from the inside out, Annette as a product innovator and Melissa as an editor and journalist. This book was propelled by our passion for beauty combined with our love of motherhood.

For both of us, entering pregnancy changed our relationship with beauty. We started taking a closer look at the personal care products we had always used and loved. Suddenly we didn't care as much about the beautiful packaging, the way they smelled, or the promises they made about evening out our skin tones and diminishing our crow's feet. We both asked a far more important question—what ingredients were in these potions anyway? From our shampoos to our lotions, our nail polish to our lipstick, we wanted our products not only to deliver results but to be safe for us and for our growing babies.

Pregnancy and motherhood is a supremely special time in every woman's life, and it shouldn't be a time fraught with anxiety and second-guessing. We put many years into writing and researching this book (while giving birth to three babies between the two of us!) so that your transition into motherhood could be less confusing and even more beautiful. To provide you with peace of mind, we've talked to some of the biggest names and brains in the worlds of beauty, skin care, and medicine; combed through hundreds of personal care products for mom and baby to find out which ones are the safest for use during pregnancy and for your baby; and screened many new ingredients as well as some that have been around for decades. The result of all this research appears at the end of each chapter and at the end of the book: comprehensive shopping lists of products we feel are the safest choices for you and your baby.

Throughout the book, you will also find invaluable tips from seasoned moms and new moms alike. Sometimes a little advice from someone who's been there is exactly what the doctor ordered! Becoming a mom changes your life in so many ways. Suddenly it's not only about you anymore—all of your decisions and purchases also affect someone else. But deciphering ingredients is no easy task, especially for anyone without a degree in science. We hope that *Belli Beautiful* will be your go-to resource when it comes to choosing personal care products for yourself and your family. We've done the legwork so you can focus on the business of being a mom.

Melissa's Story

Being a mother started the day I got the news I was pregnant. As soon as I saw the plus sign on the stick, I began making changes. I canceled dinner reservations at a sushi restaurant for the next evening, switched from coffee to herbal tea, and traded Belgian beer for root beer. But things got a little more complicated when I went into the bathroom to wash my face that night.

When you're pregnant, not every possible hazard is as black-and-white as the warnings on beer or medication labels. As a writer for leading national magazines and a former beauty editor for Sephora, I've spent the last decade testing out new lotions, creams, serums, gels, mousses, and cleansers on virtually every part of my body. I've tried every trendy new ingredient to come on the market. (Mushroom eye cream? Check. Sunscreen with goji berry? Yep. Wild rose serum? You bet.) But up until pregnancy, I never realized that some of the ingredients in these "cure-all" products might actually do more harm than good. If they made my skin look amazing and feel as soft as a baby's bottom, then what did I care? But that all changed when my baby's bottom actually started growing inside my belly.

During pregnancy, most women become hyperaware of everything they put into their bodies; I've seen many of my cautious friends go from fast-foodies to whole-foodies once they found out they were expecting. But those same friends didn't think twice about using the same health and beauty products they'd always used—not out of laziness, but out of lack of knowledge. Most of us are not aware of the potential dangers posed by the products we apply to our skin day in and day out. Many of us don't know that the ingredients in those products may get absorbed into our bloodstreams. How much gets through? That depends on the ingredient in question, how much of the body is covered by it, how long it sits on the skin, the temperature, the humidity levels, and a host of other factors, but research studies estimate that anywhere from 3 to 15 percent ends up in the bloodstream—maybe more.

I treated my pregnancy exactly like a feature story I was writing. I became an information junkie and began researching everything related to topical ingredients and pregnancy. That's when I discovered there was a name for these potentially harmful agents—*teratogens*. I had never even heard the word before.

Teratogens refer to any environmental factor—cigarettes, alcohol, medication, cosmetics—that is capable of interfering with the development of the fetus and causing birth defects. As it turns out, a whole host of the typical ingredients found in our everyday creams, lotions, and makeup are suspected teratogens. If I could increase my chances of having a healthy baby by simply making more conscious choices about what I slathered on my skin each day, then of course I would do it. What with using soap in the shower every day, washing my face twice a day, protecting my skin from the sun, and moisturizing my lips, eyes, elbows, knees, and hands—sometimes with different creams for each part—not to mention the weekly masks, manicures, and shaving, there were a lot of products I needed to scrutinize. I also began thinking that if other moms-to-be were armed with the same knowledge, they would do the same. All of my research and Googling led me to Belli, a pregnancy skin care line—and the only line, I discovered, that screens out any possible teratogens. I immediately ordered one of everything from the Belli product line.

I'm a tough crowd when it comes to cosmetics. Being a beauty editor has made me particularly discerning when it comes to product formulations. And I'm not a prestige snob either. I've been known to toss $200 jars of cream in the trash if they left even a trace of stickiness on my skin. So after my Belli products arrived and I had tried them out, I did something I had never done before—I reached out to Belli's founder, Annette Rubin, to tell her how impressed I was with her products. We immediately got into a conversation about how little truthful information was disseminated about topical product safety during pregnancy and nursing. We agreed that the overwhelming amount of noise about organic beauty products, which trumped everything else when it came to being a safe, conscious consumer, was misleading. When Annette told me that many of the ingredients found in the average personal care product were linked to birth defects (around 20 percent!), I knew something had to be done. Annette's research had to get out there and be more easily available. That was when the idea for this book was born.

Annette's Story

I was so happy to discover that I was expecting my first child. Knowing that big changes were on the way, I anxiously examined my daily habits to see which ones could stay and which ones I would need to do away with in order to create the healthiest possible environment for my baby. Immediately, I kicked the caffeine habit and saw a dietitian, who helped me plan daily meals that would give me optimal nutrition. Confident in my healthy new routines, I was taken aback when I read an article about the controversy over whether pregnant women should color their hair.

If hair coloring is so controversial, I immediately thought, *wouldn't all the topical skin care products I use daily also be controversial?* After all, I only colored my hair every eight weeks, but I used dozens of personal care products every day, all throughout the day. My morning routine included a plethora of hair, skin, and body care products as well as color cosmetics. I washed and moisturized my hands and reapplied lip gloss throughout the day and didn't hit the pillow at night until my evening skin care rituals were completed: applying another series of cleansing, toning, and moisturizing products for meaningful beauty sleep. It seemed to me that the debate shouldn't be just about hair color, but about a larger question: are the ingredients that pregnant women put on their skin each day potentially harmful to their unborn babies?

I took this question to my husband, who happens to be a physician. His response startled me—he said that topical skin care ingredients can be absorbed into the bloodstream, and he assumed that all skin care companies screen out ingredients linked to birth defects. But as a veteran of the beauty industry, I knew the truth—skin care companies don't talk about safety during pregnancy, and most won't even admit that topical absorption happens.

I had spent most of my life in the beauty industry, starting at the age of fourteen selling Avon to friends, family, and neighbors. I paid my way through college working behind a Clinique counter. I worked my way up the corporate ladder and eventually held executive positions at May Companies and Estee Lauder Companies. Having earned my stripes, I knew that the beauty industry is not tuned in to safety concerns during pregnancy, nor has it invested in the resources that would lead to greater understanding of the internal impact of externally applied products.

My husband and I immediately felt compelled to research the subject and learn more. It turns out that there is about a 3 percent chance of having a baby with a birth defect; this is called the *background risk*. Medical research has uncovered the reasons behind some of these birth defects, but in 70 percent of cases the cause is still unknown; scientists suspect that exposures to chemicals in our environment are part of the problem. Next we wondered whether the ingredients in everyday skin care products are linked to birth defects. Perhaps they could be contributing to this other 70 percent? So we decided to take a look. What we found was shocking.

Around 20 percent of the ingredients in most personal care products have some links to birth defects or miscarriage in published medical studies.

In response, we founded Belli in 2002—the only skin care company in the world that thoroughly reviews the medical research and eliminates questionable ingredients during pregnancy.

It wasn't long before Belli's loyal users were coming to us for our opinion on postpregnancy skin care concerns as well. They wanted advice on how to treat stretched skin, slackened skin, dark circles around the eyes from lack of sleep, and chapped skin that was causing nursing discomfort. After listening to them carefully, we studied the ingredients of skin care products to find ones that would work safely to treat these issues.

We found that the ingredient safety profile for the expecting mom is different from the profile for the nursing mom. Certainly both profiles are very different from what we need—and more importantly, need to avoid—in personal care products for babies. We knew that the LACTMED (Drugs and Lactation) database would help rule out ingredient no-nos for the nursing mom and that estrogen-mimicking ingredients (xenoestrogens) should be avoided in infant and child skin care. We used this information to create and launch two new line extensions, Belli Motherhood and Belli Baby, in 2007.

I strongly feel that all women should be informed of any possible harm they might be exposing themselves to during pregnancy and nursing—especially when it involves products that are so interwoven in our everyday lives. This book allows us to share some of the research we uncovered while creating the entire Belli line.

Though Belli continues to grow, the company doesn't yet have a product for every personal care and beauty concern. We're still often asked: *Which shampoos should I use? Which deodorant or toothpaste? What about makeup?* To address these additional questions and to help moms-to-be make the smartest product choices, we've now done safety reviews of other brands' health and beauty products and can recommend some other products as well as the ones we created. You will find all of these recommendations in the chapters of this book.

Motherhood is a full-time, forever job. With this book, my hope is to give new moms the tools they need to be as safe, informed, and confident in their choices as they can possibly be.

How to Use This Book

During our first pregnancies, we both spent a lot of time on the Internet (as most moms-to-be can relate to), Googling everything from morning sickness cures to nursery color schemes. As anyone who searches the Web for answers to questions will tell you, there is a lot of conflicting information out there. Pregnancy is not a time when you want to get your advice from a random, uninformed source. If you search online, you will find many sources telling you that topical absorption isn't something to worry about, but as we explain later, that is untrue. If there is ever a time to start thinking about the safety of the chemicals you are exposed to, it's during pregnancy. In a 2004 study called "Body Burden—The Pollution in Newborns" conducted by the Environmental Working Group, umbilical cord blood was tested in ten newborns from across the country.[1] An average of 200 industrial chemicals and pollutants, including pesticides, industrial by-products, and mercury were found. In fact, the tests showed that the newborns had 287 combined chemicals in total. Among the chemicals detected, 208 have been linked to birth defects or abnormal development in animal studies. Although the study looked only at industrial chemicals, we feel that exposure to questionable ingredients anywhere—whether they are in the air, the water, or our beauty products—should be avoided. It can be hard to control the chemicals we breathe in, but we can at least control the chemicals we apply to our skin.

Our goal in this book is not to scare you, but to make you aware that you have choices when it comes to your beauty and personal care regimen during pregnancy. You can stay with your status quo products, you can go "au natural" and use nothing at all, or you can make a third choice—switch to products that avoid potentially harmful ingredients. We don't expect anyone—including ourselves—to give up the products that make them feel and look good, but we do think that we can make smarter choices during these crucial nine months of development.

As the world becomes a smarter place, we're finally waking up to the fact that harmful chemicals are turning up in everything from our water bottles to our skin care products. But we can make certain choices about the products we buy and use. We may not be able to control every potentially harmful chemical being manufactured, but we can control what we put on our bodies. Just as you will undoubtedly baby-proof your house when your bundle arrives, we think baby-proofing your body during pregnancy is just as important, if not more so. The growth of just a few cells into a full-grown, healthy person with functioning organs and muscles is a miraculous example of Mother Nature at work, and it's not something we want to mess with by adding potentially harmful chemicals to the mix.

We're the first ones to admit that we wouldn't feel like ourselves if we didn't use the right mix of soap, moisturizer, foundation, and sunscreen every day, and the months when we were pregnant were no exception. Therefore, we've worked hard to find products from brands across the board—mass and prestige, natural and traditional—that we'd be comfortable using on our own bodies during pregnancy. Not only will we share those products with you in this book, but we also want to teach you how to be on the lookout for certain ingredients so you can make smart decisions on your own. And isn't trying to make smart decisions for ourselves and our families what motherhood is all about?

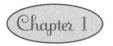
Healthy Beauty for
a Healthy Pregnancy

I f you're like us, you have been imagining for many years what you will look like pregnant. Both of us had a vision that looked something like a rosy-cheeked, Botticelli-esque beauty with added voluptuousness in all the right places. And for both of us, when the time came to actually bear a child, that aesthetic ideal fell a little short. We both dealt with bouts of acne, Melissa suffered from dermatitis (dry, itchy patches of skin in weird places on her face and body), and Annette unexpectedly gained weight in her legs first. So the truth is, just as you can never predict how long it will take you to get pregnant, you can never anticipate the beauty challenges that will come your way during gestation. And if you have more than one child, you're likely to discover that those challenges vary from one pregnancy to the next.

Thankfully, there are countless products on the market that can help you look and feel a whole lot better, regardless of the state your body is in. But here's the tricky part: just as you're so careful about what you put *in* your body during pregnancy, you need to be just as cognizant of what goes *on* your body.

You may think that applying a skin cream or eye shadow is perfectly safe for the growing baby inside your belly, but unfortunately, thanks to topical absorption, that's not always the case. *Topical absorption* happens when some of the ingredients you apply to your skin get into your bloodstream, where they can affect the little person you're working so hard to protect. Thus, even as you're being so careful about your diet, your favorite hand lotion, which you may apply three times a day, may actually be exposing your baby to harmful chemicals.

Are you devoted to natural and organic products? If so, you may be thinking, *Since I'm so careful to use only products that claim to be good for me and good for the environment, they must be safe for my baby as well.* This kind of thinking is completely logical, but unfortunately it's also completely false. In this chapter, we explain why.

It would also be logical to wonder: *Why, if these ingredients are potentially harmful, are they even available for the public to buy and use?* The answer is that the US Congress did not give the Food and Drug Administration (FDA), the body that regulates cosmetic products, the mission of reviewing the safety of cosmetic ingredients before they are put on the market. According to the agency's website, the "FDA's legal authority over cosmetics is different from other products regulated by the agency, such as drugs, biologics, and medical devices. Cosmetic products and ingredients are not subject to FDA premarket approval authority, with the exception of color additives."[1] The agency clearly states that each manufacturer has the responsibility of ensuring the safety of its own products. There may be one or more studies showing links between a cosmetic ingredient and birth defects in animals, but the research is either missed or ignored by the companies that make the products. It can be years or decades before the FDA or some other regulatory agency takes action because it can take that long before an ingredient is finally proven to be harmful in multiple human studies.

This means that the beauty industry—a $50 billion industry—was intended to be primarily self-regulated. In 1976 a self-regulating committee called the Cosmetic Ingredient Review (CIR) panel was formed by the Personal Care Products Council, a cosmetics industry trade group. The CIR "reviews and assesses the safety of ingredients used in cosmetics in an open, unbiased, and expert manner, and publishes the results in the peer-reviewed scientific literature."[2] That may sound like a good deal, but not everybody agrees. According to the Campaign for Safe Cosmetics, the CIR

> operates in a vacuum of guidance from FDA when it comes to the safety of personal care products. Words on labels like "natural," "safe" and "pure" have no definition in law and no relationship to the hazard inside the packaging. Acceptable levels of risk are entirely at this panel's discretion. To the detriment of public health, the CIR doesn't look at the effects of exposures to multiple chemicals linked to negative health impacts; the cumulative effect of exposures over a lifetime; the timing of exposure, which can magnify the harm for the very young and other populations; or worker exposures, in both beauty salons and manufacturing plants.[3]

This means that consumers—especially pregnant women—need to be their own ingredient scouts. Not an easy feat considering how many ingredients and chemicals there are in the products on the market and how confusing their names are. In this book, we will help you sort them out so that you can pinpoint the teratogens and better understand what you should be avoiding during pregnancy. We will also tell you which ingredients make for safer choices.

At this point you may also be thinking: *If I only use a few products each day, can they really make that much of an impact?* The answer is, yes they can. Although there may be only trace amounts of the bad stuff in each of your products, they can add up and accumulate in your body over the years. This is something that filmmaker Penelope Jagessar Chaffer discovered firsthand during the making of her documentary *Toxic Baby,* which investigates the effects of everyday chemicals on our children. Jagessar Chaffer interviewed scientists and doctors from prestigious hospitals and universities all over the world on the topic of environmental chemical exposure. She also got her own blood tested for the film, to see what chemicals turned up. The test revealed a large amount of PCBs (polychlorinated biphenyls), chemicals used in electric motors, in her system. The surprising part? Legislation banning the use of PCBs was introduced in the 1970s. Jagessar Chaffer also found out that her blood bore a large amount of *phthalates,* which are found in many beauty products; for instance, phthalates are the main component of fragrances. Their presence is very hard to decipher from the ingredients list on your product package, but we will tell you more about how to decode this ingredient in the next chapter.

Understanding Topical Absorption

We believe that motherhood begins the second you see the plus sign on the pregnancy test. Once you see that sign, everything changes. You are now responsible for the health and well-being of another human being. Quite a daunting thought, if you ask us. Nevertheless, there is no better time to clean up your act in the health and beauty department than when you find out you're a mom. We both gave up many of our daily vices, like coffee, red wine, Diet Coke, and Twizzlers. We tried to stay away from foods with artificial additives and ate as many veggies and fruits as we could stomach (not easy when you've got morning sickness). As babies grow they depend on their moms for the vitamins and minerals critical to development, so we both took prenatal supplements with DHA (an omega-3 fatty acid) to ensure that our little ones got all the nutrition they needed.

While most pregnant women are well aware of how important it is to try to eat healthy, it's the other environmental factors that are a little harder to understand. At your first prenatal checkup, your doctor, like most obstetricians, will probably hand you a list of forbidden foods but never mention the potential hazards of the topical products women use every single day. "The OB is usually so busy that they don't have a chance to talk about it or there's a lack of knowledge," says perinatologist Dr. David Abel. He's right. It's easy to think that the creams or lotions we put on our skin are not doing much to us beyond affecting only the top layer. But the truth is that our skin is not a perfect barrier.

The topical ingredients we apply to our skin are absorbed into our bodies through several routes. Some enter through the hair follicles and sweat glands. Some diffuse along the cells of the epidermis, then through the skin's basement membrane and into the dermis, where the tiny capillaries are located. Absorption can also occur through cuts, scrapes, or breaks in the skin—and not just through large lacerations but through micro-abrasions and sunburns as well. In other words, absorption can happen anywhere the skin has broken down and lost some of its defenses. The temperature also plays a part in the absorption rate. Heat and humidity increase the rate of absorption, as does exercise, which dilates our blood vessels and opens up our pores. Over time, these topical exposures can add up. In fact, just looking at the effects of topical products like nicotine patches, heat rubs, and some birth control patches will make you realize that what we put on our bodies does indeed affect us internally.

Everything you eat, drink, breathe, touch, and apply also has the potential to affect your unborn baby—and not just the skin cream you used today, but the products you used yesterday and the day before. "The problem is that we collect so many of these chemicals throughout our lives," says Jagessar Chaffer. "Many of these toxins are just sitting in the fat reserves in our bodies, and when we become pregnant our bodies start breaking down those fat reserves to fuel the very rapid changes and growth going on with the embryo and fetus." Once the fat reserves break down, the chemicals they stored are released into the bloodstream and can potentially affect any organ or function in the human body. And because the poorly named "placental barrier" is actually more of a widely spaced filter, those chemicals can cross into the unborn baby's bloodstream. The placental barrier blocks very large particles, such as bacteria, but allows most of the smaller chemicals to pass through. (It's unclear exactly which chemicals cross the placental barrier, or in what amounts, as researchers avoid drawing blood from human fetuses.) "Our placentas have not evolved over time to deal with all of these new chemicals," says Jagessar Chaffer. "The placenta will take waste out, but the waste products it is used to dealing with are from our blood or bodily fluids. It doesn't know what to do with the ingredients from your lipstick or skin cream."

Sure, those chemicals can have an effect on me as an adult, you may be thinking, *but my organs are already formed, unlike those of my developing baby. If it's too late to do anything about the many chemicals already stored in my system, what's the harm of adding more?* That kind of thinking is very dangerous. As Jagessar Chaffer points out in her film, our bodies contain 30,000 to 50,000 chemicals that our grandparents did not have in their bodies, simply because they had not been invented. New chemicals, including topical ingredients, are being produced every year. Which ones will have an effect on fetuses? In what amounts? These questions are difficult to answer with any certainty, and that's why it's so important to be mindful of the ingredients you're putting on your body during pregnancy, as well as the ingredients you use once your baby is born.

At that point, with your baby out in the real world, you face a whole other set of choices. As any new mom who's stepped inside one of those multifloor baby emporiums knows, there are literally thousands of baby products to choose from. It can be very tempting to buy something because the packaging on the bottle matches your nursery room decor or because the fragrance mimics that new baby smell. But the truth is that, as parents, we have to be careful about what we put on our little ones' skin. In children and infants, the reproductive system is still developing and maturing, and they are very sensitive to higher levels of estrogens or *xenoestrogens*— chemicals that mimic the effects of estrogen in the human body. In newborn males, estrogen exposure has been linked to abnormal breast enlargement, decreased sperm counts, and decreased testosterone levels. In females, scientists speculate, exposure to xenoestrogens in the environment may explain the earlier onset of puberty so common in girls today.

Sadly, many of the beautifully packaged baby products on the market are formulated with a whole host of no-no ingredients. Soy, an ingredient found in many baby formulas, is thought to be a xenoestrogen. A few case reports suggest that lavender, an ingredient used in tons of baby care products because of its soothing fragrance, also has estrogenic effects. Products containing parabens and phthalates are also estrogenic; you'll probably see these ingredients listed on the back of a typical baby wash or lotion.

"All of the genes in our body are regulated by hormones," explains Jagessar Chaffer. "Hormones will tell a gene when to turn on and when to turn off." All of the hormone-mimicking chemicals behave like real hormones, and it is when they switch genes on and off that certain disorders can occur. The bottom line is this: because topical absorption could allow the ingredients in health and beauty products to affect the development of the baby forming inside our body as well as the baby's development once the child is born, we have to be vigilant about what we put on our and our children's skin.

Understanding Teratogens

What does "teratology-screened" mean exactly? *Teratology* is the study of chemicals that cause birth defects. *Screening* is a process of examining a group of items very carefully to exclude any undesirable elements. When Belli creates products for their pregnancy collection, their physicians search through millions of published medical studies to make sure no links have been reported between any of the ingredients and birth defects or miscarriage, in either animal or human studies, at any dose, or through any method of absorption. Belli applies these criteria of teratology screening because they assume that, no matter how a chemical is absorbed, it still eventually reaches the shared maternal-fetal bloodstream.

Belli's teratology screening includes searches of the MED-LINE, TOXLINE, DART, TERIS, and REPROTOX databases, which contain over 15 million articles in over 5,000 international journals. They also use several standard teratology reference books: *Catalog of Teratogenic Agents, Drugs in Pregnancy and Lactation: A Reference Guide to Fetal and Neonatal Risks,* and *Chemically Induced Birth Defects.*[4] The process can take months to complete for every ingredient. For this book, we have used a more streamlined version of this approach to screen thousands of ingredients in hundreds of beauty products on the market today.

Since it's unethical to do any kind of testing on a pregnant woman, most teratology research has been based on animal studies. Belli does not perform animal testing itself, but instead looks at existing animal research to help determine which ingredients are the safest. Belli also looks at research on women whose babies were born with birth defects to determine the cause of the birth defect. In this kind of "retrospective" research, conversations and interviews are used to try to pinpoint the teratogen.

The US FDA Pregnancy Risk System

Another example of using teratology research to evaluate safety is the Food and Drug Administration's Pregnancy Risk Classification System. Created in 1979, this system assigns prescription and over-the-counter medications to different categories (A, B, C, D, and X). The hope at the time was to help doctors and patients make better risk decisions about which treatments to use during pregnancy. The categories weren't intended for use with cosmetic ingredients because back in 1979 most people thought that skin care products didn't enter the body.

One simple way to think about Belli's teratology screening process is that it would exclude any chemicals classified as category C, D, or X.

Category A: Adequate and well-controlled studies have failed to demonstrate a risk to the fetus in the first trimester of pregnancy (and there is no evidence of risk in later trimesters).

Category B: Animal reproduction studies have failed to demonstrate a risk to the fetus and there are no adequate and well-controlled studies in pregnant women.

Category C: Animal reproduction studies have shown an adverse effect on the fetus, and there are no adequate and well-controlled studies in humans, but potential benefits may warrant use of the drug in pregnant women despite potential risks.

Category D: There is positive evidence of human fetal risk based on adverse reaction data from investigational or marketing experience or studies in humans, but potential benefits may warrant use of the drug in pregnant women despite potential risks.

Category X: Studies in animals or humans have demonstrated fetal abnormalities and/or there is positive evidence of human fetal risk based on adverse reaction data from investigational or marketing experience, and the risks involved in use of the drug in pregnant women clearly outweigh potential benefits.

Five Baby Steps to Safer Skin Care

Baby Step 1: Turn Yourself into an Avid Ingredients Reader

When we become pregnant, we are so careful about what we eat during those nine months of gestation—as we should be—but many of us mindlessly apply the same skin care, hair care, and makeup products that we've always used, without checking the labels for their ingredients. Even if most of us did start checking labels before applying these products, how would we even know if a product was a potential hazard to our unborn baby? This is exactly why we wrote this book—so that pregnant women and new moms can become better at recognizing which ingredients are safer than others.

Pregnancy immediately turns most women into ingredient readers—we cautiously eye the fine print on our prenatal vitamins, multigrain cereal, and favorite beverages—but deciphering the back of our face cream can be a bit trickier because the chemicals listed there are not words we come across every day. We hope that reading this book will make you just as comfortable with the words on your beauty product packages as you are with the ones on the back of your cereal box.

Since it's up to you to make your pregnancy the safest it can possibly be—no one else is going to do it for you—we want to make ingredients reading as easy as possible for you. Throughout the book, we identify, explain, and define many of the key ingredients found in both mom and baby products. Our "Choose to Use" and "Reduce Your Use" lists spell out which ingredients are okay for mom and baby and which ones are not.

It's important to keep in mind that when we talk about potentially harmful ingredients in this book, we're talking about *suspected* teratogens. There simply isn't enough research yet to be able to say that certain agents definitely cause birth defects in people. But we're not risk takers—especially where our babies are concerned. This is a case where we certainly would rather be safe than sorry.

Baby Step 2: Don't Be Fooled by the Words "Organic" and "Natural"

Millions of people today buy organic and natural beauty products in the belief that these products are not only good for the environment but also nontoxic and healthy for their body and healthy for their baby's body. It's an easy trap to fall into—*If it says "organic" on the label,* you may think, *then it must be safe.* Not so! "Organic" just means that the plant was grown without the use of any pesticides and was processed without the use of any synthetic chemicals. "Organic" says nothing about the safety of the plant itself! In fact, the FDA recently addressed this common myth: "An ingredient's source does not determine its safety. For example, many plants, whether or not they are organically grown, contain substances that may be toxic or allergenic."[5]

Some plants are safe and beneficial to humans, but not all of them are. So what exactly is it about some organic products that doesn't necessarily make them safe for pregnant women and babies? Over millions of years, many plants have acquired the ability to protect themselves from predators by producing chemicals that are toxic or poisonous. Exposure to stinging nettle, for example, causes skin pain and irritation. Poison ivy causes an allergic rash. We extract salicylic acid—an ingredient commonly used in anti-acne products—from willow tree bark, but this ingredient is also linked to birth defects and miscarriage in mice. Aloe vera has soothing and anti-inflammatory properties, but it is also linked to birth defects and fetal death in rats. These are just a few examples of natural and organic ingredients that can be harmful to living organisms—there are dozens and dozens more. This is yet another reason why deciphering the ingredients in your products is so important!

So when we hear about a skin care product—especially those targeted to babies and pregnant women—being touted for its "organic" ingredients and having all sorts of claims made about how healthy it is just because it's organic, it makes us want to scream. Marketers do an excellent job of swaying consumers to spend their money on anything with the word "organic" on the bottle. Sometimes their nontoxic claims are true, but most of the time the ingredients list is rife with many potential teratogens.

Being fooled by "organic" and "natural" claims on a product is a good example of how confusing all this can be. Just when you thought you were taking the extra step and doing the right thing for yourself and your baby, you could actually be doing the opposite.

Baby Step 3: Edit Your Beauty Routine

For us, stopping cold turkey on using beauty products during pregnancy and nursing was not a viable possibility, but neither could we keep using the same products we'd always used. In this book, we offer you a third alternative, a middle ground somewhere between using no products at all and making no changes in your beauty regimen.

Think of your pregnancy as a nine-month beauty diet. Start by cutting back on some of the potentially harmful ingredients. If you find you can't live without them, use them sparingly, and never on broken skin or cuts. Remember that pregnancy and nursing do not last a lifetime. We're talking forty weeks and however many months you choose to breast-feed. You can always go back to your regular beauty routine afterward.

Neither of us would claim to be a pregnancy puritan. During our own pregnancies, we tried not to drive ourselves crazy obsessing about each and every lotion, soap, and lip product that grazed our skin. We wrote this book to help you make the safest, smartest choices you can, not to totally freak you out. We want your pregnancy and first year of motherhood to be a time of joyful wonder and happy discoveries, but we also want it to be the time when you begin making more cognizant choices with respect to the products you buy and the advice you take.

Baby Step 4: Limit Your Exposure to Potential Toxins

After you become familiar with the ingredients to avoid, the next step is either to eliminate them completely or to apply them sparingly, with some guidelines. "With drugs—especially prescription drugs—we know the dosage someone is taking for a particular condition. With cosmetics, there is no way to know how big [a] chemical dose someone is getting," says Dr. Janine Polifka, past president of the Organization of Teratology Information Specialists (OTIS). "One person might slather on a product, and one might use only a small amount." Translation: whether you apply a nickel-sized portion of skin cream versus a heaping mound may have a direct effect on your—and your baby's—safety. In addition to practicing product portion control, there are other ways you can minimize the effect of any potentially toxic ingredient:

- Never apply products to wounds, damaged skin, or sunburns.
- Don't use occlusive (nonbreathable) dressings.
- Always apply products in a well-ventilated room.
- Try to avoid all questionable ingredients, especially during your first trimester, when the fetus is in the very early growth stages. Our advice is, *when in doubt, wait it out.*

Baby Step 5: Use the Products Recommended in This Book

We combed through literally hundreds of products on the market during our research for this book. Every product we recommend has been carefully screened for links to teratogens. You may wonder if some teratogens are worse than others. The answer is, we just don't know. Since teratology research on skin care ingredients is still in its early stages and very little has been done on humans, it's not clear (1) which chemicals are worse than others, (2) what dosages are safe or dangerous, or (3) when during pregnancy a chemical becomes more safe or more dangerous. With so much uncertainty, we think it's best to try to avoid all suspected teratogens throughout your entire pregnancy. That's not an easy thing to do, but by following our product recommendations, you will certainly be limiting the amount to which you are exposed.

Belli's pregnancy skin care products all screen 100 percent clean for suspected teratogens. It is extremely hard—if not impossible—to find other products that screen completely clean because other companies aren't looking at their ingredients that way; among them, we did, however, identify some safer, smarter options. Our carefully chosen selection of recommended products screen at least 90 percent teratogen-free, which is still far cleaner than the average personal care product.

We want to make it clear that just because you have used a product with ingredients we are red-flagging in this book *does not mean* that your unborn baby has been harmed. Just as some women choose not to drink a sip of alcohol during pregnancy rather than take any risk, we are taking the same conservative approach to beauty products. Our goal with this book is to inform, not to scare. "It's very important to understand that every woman has a 3 to 5 percent chance of giving birth to a baby with a birth defect, no matter what they take or what agents they're exposed to," says Dr. Polifka. "It's extremely hard to provide the information women need to have safe pregnancies without scaring them or causing unnecessary litigation." She's right. At this point in medical research, it's impossible to trace a birth defect back definitively to a specific topical ingredient. We're giving you the best guidelines we possibly can since there is so much uncertainty out there.

You might be surprised by some of the products we're recommending in the book. Some are "natural" or "organic," but many are not. Our cosmetics wardrobe consists of products from the luxury department store, the cool downtown indie boutique, *and* the drugstore. We're equal opportunity when it comes to choosing our beauty products, and that's exactly how we went about searching for products to screen for this book. You'll find offerings from popular brands that we swear by as well as amazing products from a bunch of under-the-radar brands that we fell in love with during the writing of this book. All of them have the same thing in common—they are products we'd feel comfortable using ourselves during pregnancy—in fact, many of them we did!

Chapter 2

Ingredient Watch

Let's start out by separating fact from fiction. The last thing we want is for you to look at your jar of eye cream as if it were a bag of rat poison. Yes, there are concerning ingredients out there, some of which have ended up in our cosmetics and personal care products, but the media is just as likely to overhype things as they are to downplay them. We want you to have the correct information so you can make an informed decision about whether or not to use a product.

All cosmetic ingredients fall into different classes. Some of these classes, such as *parabens,* a family of preservatives, have become part of the popular vernacular of late, while others, such as *ethoxylated ingredients,* remain more obscure. As a new mom, what you want to know is how any particular ingredient is going to affect you and your baby, and that is exactly why we've broken it down for you in this chapter. Here's everything you need to know about all the potentially harmful classes of ingredients in personal care products and their possible impact on you during the different stages in early motherhood.

How to Read Labels

In learning how to read the ingredient lists on your health and beauty products, it's important to start with some basics. First, you should know the difference between a "cosmetic" and an "over-the-counter (OTC) drug product." According to the FDA, a cosmetic is a product (except soap) that is "intended to be rubbed, poured, sprinkled, or sprayed on, introduced into, or otherwise applied to the human body . . . for cleansing, beautifying, promoting attractiveness, or altering the appearance." A cosmetic is also a drug when it is intended "for use in the diagnosis, cure, mitigation, treatment, or prevention of disease" or intended "to affect the structure or any function of the body of man or other animals."[1] Cosmetic products list ingredients in descending order of concentration, with the highest percentage concentration appearing first on the list. For ingredients with a concentration of 1 percent or less, companies can add them to the bottom of the list in any order they want. With an OTC drug product, the active ingredients appear in a drug fact box, along with uses, warnings, and directions. The inactive ingredients in an OTC product are listed last, usually in alphabetical order.

Class: Parabens

How Parabens Appear on Labels

There are four parabens found most often in personal care products:

- Methylparaben
- Ethylparaben
- Propylparaben
- Butylparaben

You will sometimes see them grouped together like this:

* Paraben (methyl, ethyl, propyl, butyl)

Less common forms of parabens include:

* Isopropylparaben
* Isobutylparaben
* Benzylparaben

Why Parabens Are in Your Products

Any cream, lotion, or gel that features water as an ingredient is prone to bacterial contamination. (Pure oils are immune.) Chemists add preservative ingredients to kill bacteria so that the product will remain fresh and clean—even after it's been stored on a shelf or in your medicine cabinet for several years.

What You May Have Heard About Parabens

No ingredient has suffered from a worse case of bad PR than the class of preservatives known as parabens, and rightly so. All of the controversy started when high amounts of parabens were detected in the tumor cells of women diagnosed with breast cancer—especially tumors located in the upper, outer quadrant of the breast. The assumption was that parabens in deodorants and antiperspirants were getting absorbed through the armpit and somehow working their way down to the breast tissue, where they were causing the tumors. But there is another side to the story. Though parabens were found in the tumor tissue, it has never been proven that they were responsible for causing the cancer.

The Research on Parabens

Beyond the cancer controversy, research has also linked many parabens to birth defects, miscarriage, and reproductive problems:

- Subcutaneous injection of pregnant animals with butylparaben increased the rate of fetal and newborn death, decreased the body weight of newborn females, and caused reproductive system malformations in newborn males.[2]
- Oral exposure of newborn males to propylparaben decreased testosterone levels and caused dysfunction of the reproductive system. The effect occurred at a dose similar to approved propylparaben daily intake levels in the European Community and Japan.[3]
- Oral exposure of newborn males to butylparaben decreased testosterone levels and caused dysfunction of the reproductive system. The effect also occurred at a dose similar to approved butylparaben daily intake levels in the European Community and Japan.[4]
- Methylparaben, ethylparaben, butylparaben, and propylparaben were each found to compete with estrogen-binding receptors on human breast tumor cells that were sensitive to estrogen (evidence of estrogenic effects).[5]
- In a study involving yeast, methylparaben, ethylparaben, butylparaben, and propylparaben were all found to be weakly estrogenic.[6]

What Should You Do About Parabens?

Dr. Rubin: Preservatives are necessary in skin care products because they prevent contamination by mold and bacteria. Unfortunately, only a handful of effective preservatives are available, and each of them is linked to one kind of health risk or another. What's important, then, is to choose the best preservative ingredient for a particular situation. During pregnancy, when the health of the fetus matters most, you want to use products with preservatives that are free of links to birth defects or miscarriage. Some good choices include potassium sorbate, radish root ferment filtrate, ethylhexyl-glycerine, and iodopropylbutylcarbamate.

Parabens are so widely used in cosmetics that it can be difficult to avoid them. Out of all of the parabens, the best choice seems to be methylparaben, which has the least estrogenic activity and has not been specifically linked to birth defects.

Melissa and Annette: We feel that it's best to avoid parabens during pregnancy. Though we're inclined to think that conservative use of some paraben products (like your favorite drugstore brand of eye cream) is probably fine, why take the chance during pregnancy?

Class: Phthalates

How Phthalates Appear on Labels

Unlike parabens, phthalates aren't easy to decipher on the back of your shampoo bottle. Manufacturers often abbreviate them or use their chemical names. Look for the following ingredients in your products:

- DBP (di-n-butyl phthalate), DIDP (di-isodecyl phthalate), DEHP (di-2-ethylhexyl phthalate), DINP (di-isononyl phthalate), or DEP (diethyl phthalate)
- BzBP or BBP (benzylbutyl phthalate)

Most importantly, if you see the term "fragrance" on a product, be aware that phthalates may be present. The term "fragrance" covers a combination of unlisted compounds that sometimes include phthalates.

Why Phthalates Are in Your Products

Phthalates have several different functions. They are used to make plastics softer and more flexible. Combined with other ingredients in a personal care product, they act as stabilizers, emulsifiers, lubricants, and binding agents. They're also an important component of synthetic fragrances.

You'll find phthalates in many products, such as nail polishes, deodorants, perfumes, cologne, aftershave lotions, shampoos, hair gels, and hand lotions. They're also in some flooring and car products.

What You May Have Heard About Phthalates

Phthalates have been in the news because they've been detected in high levels in babies' bodies after recent topical exposures. They are considered endocrine disruptors because they mimic the body's natural estrogen.

The Research on Phthalates

An overwhelming amount of data supports the theory that environmental phthalate exposure can affect our reproductive organs and those of our children. An eye-opening report from the Breast Cancer Fund, "The Falling Age of Puberty in US Girls," cites phthalates as a cause of early-onset puberty, a condition whose countless negative consequences include a higher risk for breast cancer as well as for high-risk behaviors associated with adolescence, such as drinking, drug use, criminal activity, and unsafe sex. Here are findings from just a handful of studies from various sources:

- Young girls in Puerto Rico with prematurely developed breasts were more likely to have high levels of phthalates in their blood.[7]
- A study at Massachusetts General Hospital linked high levels of phthalates to lower sperm concentrations and impaired sperm motility (swimming ability) in humans.[8]
- A 2006 study concluded: "In recent years, evidence has accumulated that exposure to environmental components with estrogenic activity causes reproductive disorders in human populations. Epidemiological, clinical, and experimental studies have suggested that excessive exposure to estrogens and xenoestrogens during fetal and neonatal development may induce testicular developmental disorders, leading to alterations in the adult male fertility."[9]
- A 2005 study supports this finding about the impact of phthalates on the male reproductive system: "These data support the hypothesis that prenatal phthalate exposure at environmental levels can adversely affect male reproductive development in humans."[10]
- When another team of researchers looked at the effects of phthalates on the timing of puberty, their "weight-of-the-evidence evaluation of human and animal studies suggests that endocrine-disrupting chemicals, particularly the estrogen mimics and antiandrogens, and body fat are important factors associated in altered puberty timing."[11]
- DEHP given to four- to ten-week-old male rats caused testicular atrophy and a loss of spermatids and spermatocytes—significant abnormalities of the developing reproductive systems. Other forms of phthalates produced similar effects.[12]
- Short-term exposure of mice to phthalates resulted in increased weight of the uterus, which is usually associated with estrogenic activity.[13]

- Phthalates were found at elevated levels in the urine of infants who had recently been shampooed, powdered, or moisturized with baby products.[14]

What Should You Do About Phthalates?

Dr. Rubin: Based on both animal and human data, the growing consensus is that exposure to estrogenic chemicals during infancy and childhood can alter both the development and function of the reproductive system. The only question remaining is whether humans are exposed to high enough levels in the environment to be concerned. We have several reports that prepubescent boys can absorb enough topical lavender and tea tree oil through their scalps to cause breast enlargement. We know that phthalates are found in the urine of infants after recent topical usage. And we know that 96 percent of six- to eight-year-old girls have detectable levels of the sunscreen ingredient oxybenzone in their urine. While the data is not yet conclusive enough to force regulatory agencies to ban these hormonally active chemicals from skin care products, I would urge women to make safer choices for their children and avoid phthalates.

Melissa and Annette: Bottom line: while we'd rather not see phthalates in any personal care products, the most critical place to avoid phthalates is in all of your baby's products. As the science suggests, even topical exposure to xenoestrogens can cause body changes associated with early puberty. In 2009, California banned the use of phthalates in all products intended for young children. "These chemicals threaten the health and safety of our children at critical stages of their development," former governor Arnold Schwarzenegger said. We're going to agree with California on this one.

Class: Ethoxylated Ingredients
(aka Petroleum-Derived Ingredients)

How Petroleum-Derived Ingredients Appear on Labels

Here is how you can identify petroleum-derived ingredients:

- All the polysorbates
- Sodium laureth sulfate
- Triethanolamine laureth sulfate
- All ingredients with "eth" at the end of the name
- All ingredients with "PEG" in the name
- All ingredients with "oxynol" in the name
- All ingredients with "polyethylene," "polyethyleneglycol," or "polyoxyethylene" in the name

Why Petroleum-Derived Ingredients Are in Your Products

While ethoxylated ingredients may be controversial, they actually serve important functions in a personal care product, including:

- Surfactant
- Emollient
- Emulsifier
- Stabilizer
- Thickener

What You May Have Heard About Petroleum-Derived Ingredients

Any product whose name includes the word "petroleum" has most people picturing a canister of crude oil being poured into the formula. So it's no wonder that most of us assume that any product containing these ingredients is toxic and carcinogenic.

The Research on Petroleum-Derived Ingredients

The truth is that there's nothing wrong with the petroleum-derived ingredients themselves. They work very well in the formulas for personal care products, and their low cost keeps most of these products affordable. However, the process of converting petroleum into these ingredients produces trace amounts of a contaminant called 1,4-dioxane, which is thought to be a probable carcinogen. You won't find 1,4-dioxane listed on the ingredient label, and most companies don't even know it's there. In fact, one study by the Environmental Working Group (EWG) showed the presence of 1,4-dioxane in 46 percent of personal care products.[15]

What Should You Do About Petroleum-Derived Ingredients?

Dr. Rubin: There are two ways to avoid 1,4-dioxane in your personal care products. You can either (1) avoid products that contain petroleum-derived ingredients altogether, or (2) ensure that the company has taken steps to purify these ingredients and remove contaminants.

Melissa and Annette: If the thought of searching through every ingredient label makes you want to scream, another solution is to determine whether the manufacturer has vacuum-stripped its ingredients—a simple, inexpensive purifying process that removes 1,4-dioxane. Vacuum-stripping is a great solution that's endorsed by both the FDA and the Environmental Working Group. Alternatively, we've found that lanolin has the same emollient properties as petroleum, but none of the negatives.

Class: Chemical Sunscreens

How Chemical Sunscreens Appear on Labels

You'll find many different chemical sunscreen ingredients in sunblocks and other personal care products, and new ones are invented each year. A few common chemical sunscreens include:

- Benzophenones (oxybenzone, benzophenone-3)
- Cinnamates (octyl methoxycinnamate, octocrylene, cinoxate, ethylhexyl p-methoxycinnamate, octinoxate, OMC)
- Salicylates (homosalate, homomethyl salicylate, ethylhexyl salicylate, octyl salicylate)
- 4-methylbenzylidene camphor (4-MBC)
- PABA (octyl-dimethyl PABA, OD-PABA, p-aminobenzoic acid)
- Avobenzone (parsol)

Why Chemical Sunscreens Are in Your Products

Physical sunscreens (titanium dioxide, zinc oxide) work by blocking and reflecting ultraviolet rays, but their white color and pasty texture make them less than ideal for daily use—think of the white noses you see on lifeguards. Chemical sunscreens work by absorbing the ultraviolet rays instead. Consumers love them because they're both invisible and light enough to include in a cream or a spray.

What You May Have Heard About Chemical Sunscreens

It's hard to reach for a bottle of sunscreen these days without scratching your head in confusion. The FDA's new regulations, which call for clearer labeling on bottles of sunscreen, are designed to help us weed out the safe sunscreens from the ones making all sorts of false claims. The physical blocks tend to sit on the surface of the skin, while the chemical blocks are absorbed into our bodies through the skin and can even be detected in our urine. A growing amount of evidence suggests that, once inside the body, chemical sunscreens have estrogenic effects.

The Research on Chemical Sunscreens

- Oxybenzone (benzophenone-3), homosalate (homomethyl salicylate), 4-methylbenzylidene camphor (4-MBC), octyl methoxycinnamate (octinoxate, OMC), octyl-dimethyl PABA (OD-PABA): All five of these chemical sunscreens have been shown to increase the growth of breast cancer cells known to be responsive to estrogen. Three of them increased uterine weight when fed to female rats, and one (4-MBC) increased uterine weight after topical application.[16]

- Octocrylene was found to increase the growth of breast cancer cells known to be responsive to estrogen.[17]

- Avobenzone (parsol 1789): Avobenzone is one of only three sunscreen ingredients currently allowed in the European Union (along with zinc oxide and titanium dioxide). However, this ingredient degrades quickly, so its use as a sunscreen is questionable. It is sometimes combined with other sunscreens.

- PABA (p-aminobenzoic acid) showed estrogenic activity in fish, both in a petri dish and in the living organisms.[18]

- When micronized particles and nanoparticles—which are relatively new inventions—are used in the production of titanium dioxide, the physical sunscreen becomes invisible. However, the safety of these particles has not yet been established, and there is concern that their extremely small size may significantly increase their absorption into living cells.

What Should You Do About Chemical Sunscreens?

Dr. Rubin: I strongly recommend the traditional physical sunscreens (titanium dioxide and zinc oxide) to all of my patients. They offer great broad-spectrum UVA/UVB sun protection, and they're more water-resistant, less toxic to both mom and baby, and much better for sensitive skin. Some people dislike the white color, but I think it serves a useful purpose—it's obvious when you've missed a spot while applying it. That's especially important for your baby.

Melissa and Annette: When we were pregnant, we used only the traditional physical blocks, for all the reasons stated above. Even now we continue to use the physical blocks because we both have sensitive skin and the chemical sunscreens irritate our already red-prone complexions. Plus, they're known to cause skin allergies. Another big mark against chemical sunscreens is that they can cause free radicals, which lead to wrinkles. No thanks! Our advice is to forgo the chemical sunscreens and the micronized and nanoparticles during pregnancy and nursing. If you feel like the traditional physical blocks aren't as elegant and you dislike the white film they may leave on your skin, try using a tinted version instead.

The Ingredients to Watch Out For

Now that you've learned about the different classes, here's a look at the most commonly used individual ingredients and the research linking them to birth defects. Reviewing teratology reports on ingredients is not particularly pleasant reading. Again, we need to remind you that all the research discussed here is taken from animal studies, since it's unethical to perform studies on pregnant women. Obviously, you're not an animal carrying a litter of children, so you may be wondering whether this research really applies to you. Try looking at it this way: if an ingredient has been shown to be harmful to the fetus of a living being, and a product is available that does the same job but with better ingredient choices, then why take the risk and use it on yourself when you're pregnant?

You'll notice that these studies looked at both oral (swallowed) and subcutaneous (injected underneath the skin) exposures. Whether the ingredient enters the body through the mouth, the skin, or an injection, the chemicals all end up in the same place—the shared maternal-fetal bloodstream.

Just to be clear, Belli does not perform any research on animals, either directly or indirectly through hired consultants. Belli loves animals very much and is listed as a "cruelty-free" company on the website of People for the Ethical Treatment of Animals (PETA). But we also feel that it would be irresponsible and wasteful to ignore the results of animal research in the medical community. Since experiments on pregnant humans are out of the question, this is sometimes the only way we can understand the safety of different ingredients.

It is virtually impossible to compile a complete listing of every ingredient that has been red-flagged because of links to birth defects or other harmful effects during pregnancy, since the research is constantly being updated. But we think it's important for you to know the details of some of the most common ingredients and the results of teratology research on them thus far. Remember, we think it's best to avoid these ingredients during pregnancy, but if that's not possible, then you should try to reduce your use. Look out for these ingredients on your labels.

Salicylic Acid

Related to aspirin and derived from willow bark, salicylic acid has been found to cause skeletal defects in offspring after oral exposure during pregnancy.[19]

Methyl Salicylate

Also related to aspirin, and used in over-the-counter heat cream medications, methyl salicylate has been found to cause neural tube defects (such as spina bifida) in offspring—especially near the developing brain—after topical exposure during pregnancy.[20]

Retinyl Palmitate

A vitamin A derivative and an effective anti-aging ingredient, retinyl palmitate has been found to cause cleft palate in offspring after topical exposure during pregnancy.[21] Research has also shown that retinyl palmitate causes neural tube defects (spina bifida) and fetal death after a single oral dose during pregnancy.[22]

Propylene Glycol

A humectant and slip agent with useful antifreeze properties, propylene glycol has been found to increase embryonic and fetal death in offspring after intraperitoneal (injected into the abdomen) exposure during pregnancy.[23]

Benzoyl Peroxide

A common antibacterial ingredient found in over-the-counter acne treatments, benzoyl peroxide has been found to significantly decrease body weight in offspring after exposure during pregnancy.[24]

Disodium EDTA

A stabilizing ingredient in cosmetic formulations, disodium EDTA has been found to increase rates of embryonic death after intraocular (eye) exposure during pregnancy. The effect is more pronounced as the dose is increased.[25] Disodium EDTA has also been found to increase rates of embryonic death and cause significant birth defects in offspring after oral exposure during pregnancy.[26]

Aloe Vera

A natural water-binding agent with anti-inflammatory properties, aloe vera has been found to increase rates of embryonic death and cause malformations of the limbs and ribs after oral exposure during pregnancy.[27]

Rosemary

A natural antioxidant with skin-irritating properties, rosemary has been found to increase rates of fetal death after females are impregnated by males who have received the chemical orally. Fertility is also reduced in males who receive the same treatment.[28]

BHT (Butylated Hydroxytoluene)

A synthetic antioxidant used in many cosmetic formulations, BHT has been found to cause the congenital absence of one or both eyes in offspring after oral exposure prior to mating and during pregnancy.[29] BHT has also been found to decrease sleep and learning and to increase social and isolation-induced aggression in offspring after oral exposure throughout pregnancy and nursing.[30]

Dimethicone

A silicone-based lubricant and skin protectant, dimethicone has been found to increase fetal death and cause a type of clubfoot deformity in offspring after subcutaneous (injection beneath the skin) exposure during pregnancy.[31]

Sodium Lauryl Sulfate

A commonly used surfactant (foaming cleanser) in soaps and shampoos, sodium lauryl sulfate (SLS) was found to increase rates of fetal death and cause birth defects in offspring after oral or topical exposure during pregnancy.[32] Sodium lauryl sulfate has also been found to reduce fetal weight and cause toxic effects in the mother after high-dose topical exposure during pregnancy.[33] See Chapter 4 for the difference between sodium *lauryl* sulfate and sodium *laureth* sulfate.

Polysorbate 20

Derived from coconuts or fruits and used to help stabilize cosmetic formulations, polysorbate 20 has been found to cause embryonic death and severe limb defects (similar to thalidomide) in offspring after intraperitoneal (abdominal injection) exposure during pregnancy. The effect is more pronounced as the dose is increased.[34]

Ginger

A natural anti-inflammatory agent with skin-irritating properties, ginger has been found to increase rates of embryonic death after oral exposure during pregnancy.[35]

Glycolic Acid

A natural alpha-hydroxy acid derived from sugarcane and various fruits and often used in facial peels, glycolic acid has been found to decrease fetal weight and cause malformations of the ribs, vertebrae, and breastbone in offspring after oral exposure during pregnancy.[36]

Oxybenzone

An invisible sunscreen with proven absorption through the skin, oxybenzone has been found to decrease the number of live offspring after oral exposure during pregnancy.[37]

Butylparaben

A commonly used cosmetic preservative, butylparaben has been found to increase fetal death and decrease the body weight of female offspring after subcutaneous exposure during pregnancy. Decreased weight of the testicles, seminal vesicles, and prostate glands has also been shown in male offspring.[38]

Papaya

A natural exfoliant with skin-irritating properties, extracts of unripe papaya have been found to cause problems with attachment of the embryo to the inside of the uterus after oral exposure during pregnancy.[39]

Palm Oil

A natural skin softener derived from the fruit of palm trees, palm oil has been found to cause significant brain defects, eye defects, and cleft palate in offspring after oral exposure during pregnancy.[40]

Chapter 3

Mom-Smart Facial Care

Before Melissa was pregnant, she was using a cocktail of various creams, gels, and cleansers on her face. Melissa was a fearless warrior who sampled every new brand that came her way. Her motto was: "Slather first, ask questions later." Her medicine cabinet resembled a department store, and her face was its best customer. (The term "guinea pig" comes to mind.) When she found out she was pregnant, she learned quickly from Annette that if there is ever a time to be hypervigilant about what you put on your face, it's when you've got a baby growing inside your belly. Pregnancy doesn't have to include a nine-month ban on your established skin care routine, but it should begin with some real ingredient scouting. Although Melissa didn't stop using her beloved products cold turkey, she did begin to cut back on them, and eventually she weaned herself off a potpourri of less-than-healthy products.

A new skin care line seems to hit the market every day, each one making greater claims than the one before it. The skin care industry is similar to the fashion industry: you'll often notice every skin care company using the next big thing in their creams at the same time. With hundreds of new ingredients being produced and introduced to the market every year, skin care "fashion" comes and goes so quickly that most ingredients are never scrutinized for their safety. Instead of following these trends, especially when you're with child, it's essential to focus on learning exactly what you're putting on your skin—and therefore into your body.

Of course, who really has the time to investigate all of the ingredients on the back of every package to make sure they're safe? That's where we come in. We have done a great deal of research to make sure that each and every recommended product and ingredient mentioned in this chapter (and throughout the book) has been screened for safety. You'll find lists of "Reduce Your Use" and "Choose to Use" ingredients in each chapter, but we also encourage you to refer back to Chapter 2 ("Ingredient Watch") for more details.

As much as we love our products, we both agree that during pregnancy and nursing it's best to take a minimalistic approach to the daily beauty routine and personal care regimen. The math is pretty simple. With fewer products applied to your skin, and in smaller amounts, the chance of exposing your unborn baby to potentially harmful ingredients is decreased. As we told you earlier, potentially harmful chemicals can accumulate in your body even if you're using only a few products a day. It's easy to think that using an eye cream with parabens isn't doing any harm, but if you're also using paraben-laden lotion and sunscreen every day, the amount inside your body can really add up.

By using a well-edited selection of products, you'll also be giving your skin a break from any irritating chemicals that may not have bothered you before you got pregnant but now, thanks to hormones and sensitivity, leave you with red angry skin and breakouts. We can take a cue from the Europeans, who believe that less is always more when it comes to beauty. The truth is that, pregnant or not, using too many products at once can damage the skin.

Here's what we mean by a minimalistic approach to beauty:

For the face: Cleanser, moisturizer, sunblock, eye cream, and lip
   balm
For the body: Soap, lotion, sunblock, deodorant, shaving cream,
   shampoo, and conditioner

We understand—and agree—that no one should have to forgo
wearing makeup during pregnancy. Although neither of us had ever
caked on the stuff before being pregnant, both of us certainly applied concealer, mascara, and blush every day. We will cover the
dos and don'ts of makeup in Chapter 5.

When you're not pregnant or nursing, it's great to be able to ex-
periment with virtually every mask, scrub, and serum that tickles
your fancy. But when there's another person growing in your belly
or nibbling on your nipples, it's time to put the kibosh on those fun
beauty extras. Leaving a mask with questionable ingredients on
your face and letting it sink into your pores for twenty minutes is
just not a risk worth taking. If you miss that ritual too much during
those nine months, then whip up a homemade mask with egg
whites and Greek yogurt (a favorite of supermodels and beauty insiders). You'll find more healthy homemade beauty treats throughout the book. As you'll learn here, having a baby doesn't mean you
have to forgo all of your beloved beauty rituals; it's all about finding
safer alternatives during your nine months of pregnancy and for
however long you decide to nurse.

If you come across an ingredient you don't see on our lists, we
strongly encourage you to contact the product manufacturer and
see how honestly the spokesperson discusses the issue of ingredient safety during pregnancy. If this person says: "It's safe because
it's natural," or, "Oh, it's not really absorbed through the skin," without offering evidence to prove either of those claims, then we'd
suggest that you toss that product and move on to something else.

A responsible company will tell you how it researches the safety of each ingredient for pregnant users and how decisions are made about which ingredients to avoid.

Your Skin During Pregnancy:
Nine Months of Smart Skin Care Starts Here

Thanks to hormones, pregnancy physically changes your entire body, not just your waistline, and an overload of hormones is responsible for changes like acne, sensitive skin, and dryness. This starts as soon as the egg and sperm unite, when your body immediately goes into hormonal overdrive. During the first trimester, your body is surging with hCG (human chorionic gonadotropin), a hormone made by the placenta, which begins to form when the fertilized egg implants itself in the uterine lining. About seventy days into your pregnancy, the placenta ramps up production of the hormones estrogen and progesterone. In fact, women have over one hundred times more estrogen surging through their bodies during pregnancy than before they were expecting. While estrogen explains your mood swings, breast swelling, and influx of spider veins, it's also responsible for some very important fetal development, including the maturation of vital organs like the lungs and liver. Estrogen also helps to regulate progesterone, the hormonal culprit behind the most common skin complaint during pregnancy—acne.

Here's our advice on how to safely address all the major skin issues you're likely to face during pregnancy.

How to Deal with Acne

If you're like most pregnant women, acne is your number-one complaint. Your skin probably hasn't seen this kind of hormonal activity since high school. "Even if you've never had acne, or haven't had it for a very long time, don't be surprised if you see a zit, especially around the mouth and chin areas, which are more common for acne during pregnancy," says Dr. Abel. Fluctuating hormone levels make the skin's hair follicles secrete more oil (sebum), which leads to acne breakouts. This effect is commonly seen during puberty, during menstruation, and during the first trimester of pregnancy.

"There is a sizable percentage of patients who get acne flare-ups during pregnancy," says New York City dermatologist Dr. Macrene Alexiades-Armenakas. "Acne is very difficult to treat because there are so many acne medications that are not appropriate during pregnancy." Almost all of the ingredients proven effective to treat acne, including benzoyl peroxide (linked to decreased birth weight and decreased testicular weight in animal studies) and salicylic acid (linked to higher rates of fetal malformation and fetal death in animal studies), are inadvisable during pregnancy.

Benzoyl peroxide is actually considered a drug. In the Food and Drug Administration's Pregnancy Risk Classification System (see Chapter 1), benzoyl peroxide is classified as a category C, which means that animal reproduction studies have shown that benzoyl peroxide has an adverse effect on the fetus and there have been no adequate, well-controlled studies in humans.

"Acne is not a life-threatening medical disease, it's a cosmetic problem, and I think it makes more sense to avoid these questionable ingredients," says Dr. Rubin. "A risk classification system for cosmetics does not exist because there's an inaccurate assumption that cosmetics are not absorbed. If we were to classify cosmetic ingredients, most of the ones we're saying to avoid would be category Cs, with links to birth defects in animal studies."

So what can you do about your temporary, but embarrassing, case of acne? Instead of grinning and bearing it through nine pimple-filled months, you can use smarter and safer ways to clean your pores and banish breakouts. Lactic acid is an effective and smart choice during pregnancy, as are tea tree oil and sulfur-based products.

Lactic Acid

Most of the ingredients we talk about in this book are foreign substances to humans, but lactic acid is a substance already found in your body. As your cells burn energy, they create lactic acid as a normal by-product. When you're exercising and you feel your muscles getting tired, it's because lactic acid is building up in your bloodstream. So it makes sense that since we already have it in our bodies, it would be safe to use on our skin.

Because lactic acid is an alpha-hydroxy acid, it is a very effective cleanser and exfoliator and does all the stuff that salicylic acid and glycolic acid do. Another advantage of lactic acid is that it's less irritating to the skin, which is crucial during pregnancy, a time when all the hormones surging through your body make your skin super-sensitive.

Sulfur

Sulfur helps dry out oily skin. It also breaks down dead skin cells, which would otherwise clog your pores and harbor the growth of bacteria. Teratology screening has revealed no links at all between sulfur and birth defects, miscarriage, or any other harmful effects during pregnancy, in either animal or human studies, at any dose, or from any method of absorption.

Sulfur is not to be confused with sulfa, another related class of chemicals called sulfonamides (sulfa drugs), used as antibiotics in humans. During the first few weeks of a newborn's life, sulfonamides can cause an accumulation of bilirubin. The breakdown product of hemoglobin from old red blood cells, bilirubin is normally converted by the liver into bile, which then is squirted into the digestive tract to help break down food. (You can sometimes see bilirubin in your skin: it's the yellow color that appears when a bruise starts to heal.) However, an excessive amount of bilirubin in a baby's bloodstream causes jaundice—diffuse yellowing of the skin and eyes. For this reason, many obstetricians refrain from prescribing sulfa antibiotics to patients in the final few weeks of pregnancy. Many newborns still get jaundice from breast milk or other causes, but it is easily treated with light from ultraviolet lamps.

Here is why we believe sulfur is okay to use during pregnancy. First, despite the similarity of their names, there's no evidence that sulfur has the same effects as sulfa. And second, pregnancy acne tends to flare during the first trimester, not during the last few weeks before delivery when sulfonamides are avoided. Sulfur is used in several over-the-counter acne medications—look for it under "active ingredients" in the drug fact box.

Tea Tree Oil

Tea tree oil also passes teratology screening. It's a great antibacterial and has benefits similar to those of benzoyl peroxide. If you're already an avid ingredients reader, then you may have heard reports of tea tree oil being a questionable ingredient. In an article in the *New England Journal of Medicine*, researchers discussed their investigation into why three adolescent boys developed gynecomastia (the abnormal development of breasts in males). They hypothesized that the lavender and tea tree oils in their shampoos were having estrogenic effects. When the boys stopped using the shampoos, the condition improved in all three of them.

So, are these ingredients safe to use during pregnancy? We think the answer is yes. Although the amount of estrogen in the pregnant body increases by about one-hundred-fold, both female and male fetuses are exposed to this high level of estrogen in utero without any problems. Once a baby is born, however, and no longer sharing the maternal bloodstream, exposure to external sources of estrogen can interfere with normal development of the reproductive system. Therefore, we think you should avoid baby products that contain suspected xenoestrogens (more on this in our baby chapter), but feel free to use tea tree and lavender oils as a mama-to-be.

Prescription for Acne: A Note from Annette

I've battled acne since fifth grade. I wish I could say that the fight is over, but the fact is that I'm still trying to combat it in my forties. Here are what I consider the most important tips when it comes to winning the fight against acne:

1. Wash your face religiously morning and night.

Use tepid water, cleanse with your hands, and be diligent about rinsing away *all* of your cleanser. (I rinse five times.) It took us three years of research and development to create Belli's Acne Cleansing Facial Wash, and it was worth the wait. It features lactic acid and a bit of lemon (a natural antiseptic), along with ingredients known to help reduce inflammation. It's my product of choice, and I often use it with a Clarisonic brush for daily deep cleaning.

2. Stop picking and start treating.

I get it—you want to pick, dig, squeeze, and destroy the breakout. I'm guilty too, and though I know it's the biggest acne no-no, sometimes I can't control myself. But every time I pick I'm left with a minor discolored scar on my face that can take months to fade. So I've replaced that bad zit-zapping habit with a good one—spot treating. And to counter the frustration of having a huge zit and not being able to do anything about it because you're pregnant, we've created a spot-treating product that is totally safe to use during pregnancy. Belli's Acne Clearing Spot Treatment contains the superhero ingredients sulfur and tea tree oil to safely banish breakouts during pregnancy. As we mentioned, both of these ingredients pass teratology screening and are effective in healing existing blemishes and preventing flare-ups. Another option for spot treating is a dab of tree tea essential oil on the offending spot.

3. Don't overmoisturize.

If you're experiencing breakouts, your skin is most likely producing more oil than usual, and adding more oil to acne-ridden areas may make matters worse. Moisturize only the areas on your face that are not breaking out and that feel tight and dry. Look for a lightweight hydrator that adds a boost of water to the skin and not a lot of oil—it will make your skin feel more comfortable. Another benefit is that well-hydrated skin looks healthier too.

What You Need to Know About Vitamin A

You've probably heard some warnings about vitamin A use during pregnancy. After all, Accutane, the acne drug known to cause birth defects if taken during pregnancy, is a naturally occurring derivative of vitamin A. Is vitamin A safe to use in your skin creams?

Since it's nearly impossible to know the exact amount of vitamin A you take in on a daily basis (through food and prenatal vitamins as well as skin creams), we think it's best to cut down on your topical intake of it. Here's what Dr. Rubin has to say:

"Vitamins are essential nutrients. Everybody needs vitamin A—even pregnant women. That's why you'll see it included in the standard prenatal vitamin that your doctor prescribes. But it turns out that there's a certain range you want to stay within. Being too low in vitamin A can actually cause birth defects, while too much vitamin A is strongly linked to birth defects as well. You already get a certain amount of vitamin A from the food you eat (mainly green, leafy vegetables). Prenatal vitamins are designed to supplement this amount, but they don't consider the additional sources of vitamin A you might be getting from skin care products. That's why it's best to cut down on your use of topical vitamin A ingredients during pregnancy. The two most common vitamin A derivatives in skin care and cosmetics are retinol and retinyl palmitate. Since there's a wide range of doses that could be absorbed through the skin, it's best to play it safe and avoid them."

Clear Skin Starts from Within!

Drink water and lots of it—your skin will thank you for it. We are big believers in the "you are what you eat" mantra. There's no better time to start incorporating a mega-healthy diet of whole grains, fruits and veggies, and pregnancy-approved sources of omega-3s than when you're expecting. You will quickly notice a clearer, more vibrant complexion—from head to toe!

How to Deal with Dry Skin

During pregnancy, your growing baby needs to "borrow" many of your bodily fluids to develop properly. You've probably noticed how thirsty you are these days. One of the side effects of dehydration is a loss of moisture in the skin, which leads to dryness. When the skin gets severely dry, it can crack, something you really want to avoid during pregnancy. As we mentioned before, tears and cracks in the skin allows a clear path for topical ingredients to enter the bloodstream. Later on in the pregnancy, the stretching skin of your expanding tummy may feel ridiculously itchy.

Thankfully, there are safer ways to treat dry, tight, itchy skin during pregnancy. Here's our advice.

Annette's Prescription for Dry Skin

During the first trimester, one-third of women experience oily and breakout-prone skin, one-third don't notice any difference in their skin, and the last third find their skin getting drier and drier, begging for something to replace the lost moisture. If your skin is dull, tight, and dry, try these tips:

- Cleanse using a mild cleanser and rinsing with tepid water. Choose a cleanser that has gentle, pregnancy-friendly exfoliants (lactic acid) to help dislodge the dead surface skin cells that can muddy a complexion.
- After cleansing, pat your skin dry and immediately follow with a moisturizer.
- If you're a dry skin type, use a physical exfoliant about twice a week. I love Belli's Fresh Start Pre-Treatment Scrub. Its grainy beads polish away dull skin, revealing the renewed fresh skin that lies beneath.
- For a simple and deeply moisturizing face mask, mix half an avocado with a teaspoon of sweet almond oil. Avocado is rich in vitamins, and sweet almond oil is an excellent emollient. Together they make even the driest skin feel more comfortable

and give it a luminous healthy glow. Use this mask once a week to keep your skin supple.

Annette's Favorite Pregnancy-Approved Skin Mask

I started making this mask as a teenager, since my skin was extremely oily and prone to break out. Now that my skin has become more of a combination type, I add a bit of extra virgin olive oil and honey. It truly works wonders on a dull complexion!

Combine the following ingredients:

- $1/3$ cup oatmeal (to absorb excess moisture—use oatmeal *only* if your skin is combination or oily and skip it if your skin is dry)
- $1/2$ teaspoon (for oily skin) to 1 tablespoon (for dry skin) extra virgin olive oil
- 1 egg (brightens and gives a temporary lift to the skin by tightening it [the egg white] and adding nutrients [the yolk])
- 1 tablespoon honey (helps the mask adhere to your face and may also have antibacterial properties)

Apply the mask after cleansing your face and leave it on for fifteen to twenty minutes. Rinse the mask off with lukewarm water.

Kick the Caffeine—in Your Skin Care

You probably already know that cutting down on your caffeine consumption is a good idea during pregnancy. But you may not know that caffeine can also be found in your skin care products. Many cosmetic companies use caffeine in their products because, as an antioxidant, it has anti-aging effects. And topical caffeine can be detected in the bloodstream in as little as five minutes, with peak absorption occurring by one to two hours.[1] Even though it's thought to be safe to have one cup of coffee a day during pregnancy, drinking more than 200 milligrams might have harmful effects. A study in the January 2008 *Journal of Obstetrics and Gynecology* found that pregnant women who consumed more than 200 milligrams of caffeine a day had twice the risk of miscarriage as the women who consumed no caffeine at all.[2]

Not sure what 200 milligrams of caffeine looks like? Here is the caffeine content of some everyday products:

- Starbucks coffee, grande (16 ounces)—550 milligrams caffeine
- Starbucks coffee, tall (12 ounces)—375 milligrams caffeine
- Starbucks coffee, short (8 ounces)—275 milligrams caffeine
- Brewed tea (180 to 480 milliliters)—26 to 120 milligrams caffeine
- Coke (12 ounces)—46 milligrams caffeine
- Mountain Dew (12 ounces)—54 milligrams caffeine
- Red Bull energy drink (8.3 ounces)—76 milligrams caffeine
- Monster Energy (16 ounces)—160 milligrams caffeine
- Two Excedrin tablets—130 milligrams caffeine

Since it's impossible to find out exactly how many milligrams of caffeine are being absorbed from your cream or lotion, we think it's best not to use any topical products with caffeine as an ingredient—especially if you are allowing yourself a caffeinated beverage every day.

Lip Service

Moisture loss also travels to the lips during pregnancy, so it's no wonder that constantly dry lips are a common pregnancy complaint. Lip products can be tricky, however, especially during pregnancy.

Not only are they absorbed through the very thin layers of the lips, but they will undoubtedly be digested too. In fact, the average woman ingests four pounds of lip product over a lifetime!

So how do you find a lip-soothing balm or ointment you can smile about during those nine months and beyond? One of the most popular cures for dry lips is any product with petroleum in it, but as you'll read in the next section, we recommend that you not use anything containing petroleum while you're pregnant unless you know it's been vacuum-stripped for purity. What can you safely use, then, to ward off chapped lips? Here are some general guidelines:

- Invest in a humidifier to replenish moisture in the air.
- Drink extra fluids to boost hydration.
- Fight the urge to lick your lips! Wetting the lips is a quick fix, but it only makes them dryer in the long run.
- When in doubt, use olive oil or lanolin (the same pregnancy-safe ingredient used in nipple creams) to soothe dry lips.

We love these pregnancy-safe ingredients for the lips:

Coconut oil smells like a day at the beach and makes our lips feel super-soft.

Beeswax, a by-product of honey production, is a common lip balm ingredient because it soothes the lips and helps heal chapping.

Shea butter is made from vegetable fats that rejuvenate the skin and lips while also protecting them from the elements, and it has major therapeutic properties.

Mango butter is an extremely soothing tropical treat for the lips. It contains natural UV protection (but you should still wear sunblock on your lips), and it helps heal sunburned skin.

Avocado oil is an amazing moisturizing tonic for the skin. Easily absorbed, it rejuvenates dry and dehydrated skin more quickly than many other ingredients.

What You Need to Know About Petroleum

If you pick up any cosmetic product—especially a lip care product—and look at the list of ingredients, the odds are you'll find several that are derived from petroleum—PEG, polyethylene, or any ingredient whose name ends in "-eth." Petroleum-derived ingredients can make a product feel smoother or cause it to "foam." The truth is that there is nothing inherently dangerous about petroleum-derived ingredients themselves; in fact, they have been approved by the cosmetic regulatory departments of every major country around the world. There is legitimate concern, however, when it comes to their purity. Petroleum is converted into usable ingredients through a chemical process known as ethoxylation. This process creates small amounts of a by-product known as 1,4-dioxane, which is a probable carcinogen and is also on California's Proposition 65 list of substances known to cause cancer or birth defects. Although 1,4-dioxane could well end up in your beauty product, it won't appear on the label.

As discussed in Chapter 2, vacuum-stripping is one possible solution. This process for separating the pure ingredients from the contaminants is endorsed by both the FDA and the Environmental Working Group: "FDA notes that 1,4-dioxane can be removed 'by means of vacuum stripping at the end of the polymerization process without an unreasonable increase in raw material cost,' . . . but such treatment would be voluntary on the part of industry," the Environmental Working Group said in 2006.[3] Unfortunately, many skin care companies either do not know about the problem or are not willing to pay extra for vacuum-stripping. As a result, many products on the shelves contain trace amounts of 1,4-dioxane, which isn't mentioned on the ingredients list. If your favorite product includes petroleum-derived ingredients, you can ask the manufacturer how it ensures the purity of the product. Otherwise, we advise avoiding petroleum-derived ingredients altogether.

How to Deal with Chloasma (aka "the Mask of Pregnancy")

There's never a more important time in your life to protect your skin from the sun than when you're pregnant. The pregnancy hormones estrogen and progesterone are thought to make the pigment-producing skin cells (the melanocytes) react more strongly to sunlight, causing dark brown splotchy areas to appear on the chin, cheeks, nose, and forehead. Known as chloasma, melasma, or "the mask of pregnancy," this condition affects up to 70 percent of all pregnant women. That's why you need to cover up and wear a broad-spectrum physical or mineral (titanium dioxide or zinc oxide) sunblock with an SPF of at least 25—even on cloudy days when you're barely outside for more than a few minutes. Chloasma fades in most women after delivery, but it can persist in up to 30 percent of cases, so prevention is definitely the best strategy.

If you have this condition, your dermatologist can recommend several topical treatments after you've delivered and are no longer nursing, such as hydroquinone, tretinoids, and chemical peels.

How Safe Is Sunscreen?

Important as it is to protect yourself from the sun at all times, navigating the tricky world of sunscreen can become even trickier when there's a bun in the oven.

Avoiding the Mask of Pregnancy: A Note from Annette

The majority of us are at risk for getting the mask of pregnancy, so use your SPF diligently *before* the dark splotches appear. And trust me, it's not like you'll wake up in the morning feeling a little chloasmatic—a full-blown case can sneak up on you quickly. For some of us, it happens in only a matter of minutes! I have a tendency to get a chloasma goatee—a blotch darkening my upper lip and extending down to my chin. Needless to say, it's not a good look. Luckily, I've been able to win the war against chloasma. On those days when I know I'll be in direct sunlight for prolonged periods of time, I apply a thicker layer of sunscreen—paying particular attention to those areas that are prone to hyperpigmentation—and then reapply every hour.

You need to be especially concerned about topical absorption with sunscreens because heat, humidity, and sun are huge culprits when it comes to opening up your pores and increasing the rate at which ingredients are absorbed into your bloodstream. Say you go to the beach and apply sunscreen all over your body. It's hot out there, you're perspiring (which opens up the pores even more), and then you're reapplying the sunscreen every two to three hours. Compare this day at the beach using sunscreen with how you use eye cream, which only goes on a small surface area, or shampoo, which gets rinsed off immediately. Kind of alarming, right? That's why it's so important to be a super-sharp ingredients reader when it comes to sun protection skin care.

There are two kinds of sunblocks: physical (mineral blocker–based) and chemical. Only use physical sunblock when you're pregnant. Teratology research shows that the physical blockers

Safe Sun Is Always in Style

The safest way to fully protect yourself from the sun is by covering up with smart and strategic accessories (we love wide-brimmed hats) and clothing. Dark-colored fabrics block out the sun better than light-colored ones, but we know how stifling it can be to wear a black T-shirt on a hot day. Our new favorite obsession is sun-protective clothing, which is made from high-tech fabrics with SPF woven into them. And since your clothing can't enter your bloodstream, they are 100 percent safe. Here are some brands to check out:

- Sun Precautions (www.sunprecautions.com): This is Dr. Alexiades-Armenakas's brand of choice. "They have amazing hats, which I basically lived in during my pregnancy," she says.
- Coolibar (www.coolibar.com): Coolibar offers everything from blouses to yoga pants fabricated out of UPF (ultraviolet protection factor) 50 sun protection.
- Cabana Life (www.cabanalife.com): Go to this site for a crisp collection of stylish, white terry-cloth beach cover-ups.
- Mott 50 (www.mott50.com): This new fashion-forward collection of tunics, wrap dresses, and basics with UPF 50 was created by two former sun-worshipers. The line is approved by the Skin Cancer Foundation, and a portion of its proceeds goes to cancer research.

(either zinc oxide or titanium dioxide) are the smarter choice over chemical sunblocks, which often include ingredients like oxybenzone or benzophenone, suspected teratogens that enter the bloodstream. The titaniums and zincs in physical sunblock sit on top of the skin and do not get absorbed. "I highly recommend physical sunblock," says Dr. Alexiades-Armenakas, who points out that the safety of chemical sunscreens has not been established.

But here's where it can get confusing. Some formulations of sunscreen contain nanoparticles of titanium dioxide and zinc oxide. Nanoparticle technology allows companies to reduce the size of those minerals so that the product goes on clear and invisible when applied to the skin rather than with the familiar white tinge. Doctors are concerned, however, that nanoparticles could be more harmful than larger forms of these ingredients. Although researchers have not established that they're dangerous, we do know that nanoparticles are much smaller than the molecules in most of the chemicals we put on our skin—and we do not know how the body handles particles that small. Are they absorbed at a faster rate? Do they enter the cells more easily? Until more is known about this new and unique kind of particle, everybody is rightfully cautious about their use during pregnancy. In fact, studies have shown that some nanoparticles are toxic to the embryos of fish.[4]

It's difficult to tell if a sunscreen was made with nanoparticles because, with their reputation, manufacturers are not advertising their use—they're just saying, "Try our great sunscreen, it goes on invisibly." Unless it says "non-nanoparticles" on the label, a product based on titanium or zinc oxide that is invisible when applied (not tinted) is probably micronized or nano. It's always better to use sunscreen than not, but personally, we'd rather smear on a sunscreen that leaves a white tinge than risk using nanoparticles, especially during pregnancy. Our advice is to cover up with sun-protectant clothing as much as possible, try to avoid the sun during the peak hours of 10:00 AM to 2:00 PM, and slather on one of the mineral (titanium dioxide or zinc oxide) sunblocks we recommend at the end of this chapter.

The Rub on Scrubs

Annette is a self-proclaimed scrub junkie who exfoliated her way through both of her pregnancies. The benefits can be immediate— softer, smoother, and more refined-looking skin with increased clarity and brightness. However, we've both learned from personal experience that an overly aggressive approach to exfoliation leaves you with dry, red, flaky, dull, irritated skin. The right amount of exfoliation is a balancing act, not a one-size-fits-all routine. Here are the basics you need to know about scrubs during pregnancy.

Regular exfoliation works by sloughing off the top layer of dead surface skin cells and revealing the healthier, younger-looking layer of fresh skin cells beneath. It also increases cellular turnover and creates a smoother, more uniform layering of the epidermis (the outer layer of skin). Freshly exfoliated skin benefits the most from the various products, such as moisturizers, whose purpose is to keep skin looking its healthiest. Treatment oils and lotions penetrate exfoliated skin more effectively and don't "lather" on top of the skin.

There are two types of exfoliation you can do at home: chemical and physical (or manual). Chemical exfoliation uses mild acids to dissolve the lipid "glue" that holds the dead surface skin cells together. These ingredients are often found in facial washes and moisturizers. Physical exfoliation uses friction from brushes, loofahs, sand, sugar, or other small granules to sweep away dead surface skin cells. Used together, physical exfoliants are more effective at removing what the chemical exfoliant has already loosened.

While pregnant, you should be particularly conscious of the type of chemical exfoliant you use. Two of the most popular exfoliating ingredients, salicylic acid and glycolic acid, have been linked to birth defects in animal studies (see Chapter 2 for details). Instead, we recommend using lactic acid, which is completely safe during pregnancy because it is already found in the body. This natural alpha hydroxy acid is very effective at exfoliation, and it also tends to be gentler and less irritating to the skin. You can use it on both your face and body—particularly if you get breakouts on your chest and back.

Annette uses a cleansing wash containing a small amount of lactic acid each morning and night and a physical grainy scrub three to four times a week to sweep away what the lactic acid has shaken loose. "I loved using a manual scrub on my abdomen when I was expecting," she says. "I would massage it in on dampened skin while in the shower, rinse it off, towel dry, and then apply a treatment oil to help prevent stretch marks on my stretching areas: tummy, breasts, thighs, hips, and buttocks. I would then moisturize all my other areas with a rich lotion. This pampering routine allowed me to care for my rapidly changing body while also connecting with my unborn baby—each time I nourished the skin on my tummy I could also feel his sweet little elbows, knees, and heels tucked up safely inside me."

Scrub Tips and Tricks

- This is one of our favorite tips, and it will help you avoid over-scrubbing. When using a manual scrub, place your thumbs under your chin and use your fingertips to gently massage your cheeks and the area around your mouth and nose. Then place a thumb on each temple and use your fingertips to gently massage the area around the orbital bone of your eye and your forehead.
- We prefer scrubs that use polyethylene micro-spheres. These beads exfoliate and polish without causing micro-tears in the skin, which could become an entry point for bacteria. If

---

Skin Smarts

- When you use a mask, peel, or anything that sits on your skin for more than a few minutes, the absorption rate goes up.
- Less is more—using less product means less absorption into the bloodstream. So think before you slather!

---

you have drier, more sensitive skin, look for scrubs in a creamier base and with fewer beads. If you are a stronger skin type that can tolerate a more assertive approach to exfoliation, look for a higher concentration of beads in a lighter-weight base.

- You can find a soft-bristled body brush if you prefer using a tool to manually exfoliate. But we don't recommend loofahs or buff puffs because they are rough on the skin, tend to exfoliate unevenly, and may cause micro-tears in the skin.

Reduce Your Use: During Pregnancy

Here's our quick list of the ingredients you should be aware of during pregnancy. For the detailed research on each ingredient, see Chapter 2 ("Ingredient Watch").

- Aloe vera
- BHT
- Butylparaben
- Dimethicone
- Disodium EDTA

- Ginger
- Glycolic acid
- Palm oil
- Papaya
- Polysorbate 20
- Propylene glycol
- Rosemary
- Sodium lauryl sulfate
- Wild black cherry

Choose to Use: During Pregnancy

- Allantoin
- Avocado (*Persea gratissima*) oil
- Beeswax
- Evening primrose
- Glycerin
- Grapeseed oil
- Jasmine oil
- Lactic acid
- Lavender
- Olive oil
- Rose hip oil
- Shea butter
- Sunflower seed oil (*Helianthus annuus*)
- Sweet almond oil
- Tea tree oil
- Titanium dioxide/zinc oxide
- Tocopherol (vitamin E)
- Vitamin C

Pregnant Pause

Ask Josie Maran,
Model/Actress/Cosmetics Entrepreneur/Mom

Q: *What lifestyle changes did you make when you found out you were pregnant?*

A: Being pregnant with my daughter Rumi Joon definitely made me more aware of what I was putting inside my body and on my skin. It made me even more adamant about not using any products that contain parabens, petrochemicals, or synthetic fragrances. I also changed my diet. When cooking, I try to use as many organic ingredients as possible and then throw all food waste into a bucket designated for compost. With a compost, you can have homegrown soil for your garden and feel good about reducing and reusing waste. Today I find other ways to make my home as eco-friendly as possible. My daughter loves getting messy, so I deal with stains all the time. But instead of bleach, I use citrus on a stain. Just rubbing and rinsing a stain with a lemon or lime, followed by a little drying time in the sun, actually does the trick.

Q: *How did you change your beauty routine during pregnancy?*

A: I paid closer attention to labels and was sure to only use products that contained natural, healthy, and nontoxic ingredients, because I knew that what you put on your body gets absorbed into the skin. After spending years in the makeup chair as a model, I enjoyed simplifying my beauty routine and going natural, just showing off my pregnancy glow!

Q: *What were your favorite products during pregnancy?*

A: It was perfect that I was pregnant while I was developing my cosmetics line. I was learning more and more about eco-friendly ingredients and using them to create some of my favorite makeup products. Of course, one of my favorite products during my pregnancy was argan oil, and it's still my favorite today. With vitamin E and essential fatty acids, it's 100 percent pure, organic, nourishing, and so moisturizing. I use it as a daily moisturizer morning and night.

Q: *What did you find to be the most successful products in making yourself look and feel good during pregnancy and those early motherhood months?*

A: Actually, eating and drinking healthy foods and beverages made me feel the best. I ate lots of organic grains, fresh fruits, and juices. And I did a *ton* of prenatal yoga. Those things and argan oil on my belly to help avoid stretch marks really did the trick!

Q: *How has motherhood changed your attitude toward health and beauty?*

A: Now that I'm a mom and have another life to protect and nurture, I make sure that what we eat as a family is really healthy. Good food is so important. In terms of beauty—just seeing my daughter smile makes me realize that being happy is the ultimate tool for looking great!

Q: *As a busy mom, what are your tried-and-true time-saving beauty secrets?*

A: I always look for multitasking beauty products with nourishing, natural, and beneficial ingredients. I love my new Argan Color Sticks—hydrating balm with 100 percent pure organic argan oil and rosy color. Two birds, one stone! Plus, you can use it on your cheeks as a creamy stick blush. It saves time and space in my makeup bag.

Q: *What's the best product from your line for creating a pregnancy glow?*

A: Argan oil! It's my beauty secret, and the one product that makes my skin glow every day. I used it during my pregnancy, and it helped to balance my complexion as my body was going through so many changes.

Q: *What's your favorite Josie Maran product for time-starved moms and moms-to-be?*

A: Argan oil again! Sense a pattern? It's my number-one favorite product simply because it's 100 percent natural and can be used for so many purposes. From a daily moisturizer to a cure for split ends, and a healing treatment for skin conditions such as psoriasis and eczema, argan oil is a multitasking cure-all that should be in every mom's makeup bag.

Mom-Safe Facial Care Product Picks

Cleansers

- Ole Henriksen African Red Tea Foaming Cleanser
- Tata Harper Regenerating Cleanser
- Burt's Bees Radiance Daily Cleanser with Royal Jelly
- Intelligent Nutrients Anti-Aging Cleanser
- Goldfaden Daily Cleanser
- bareMinerals Skincare Purifying Facial Cleanser
- Embryolisse Purifying Milk Wash
- Origins Checks and Balances Frothy Face Wash
- Duchess Marden Damascena Crème Cleanser
- Belli Acne Cleansing Face Wash
- The Organic Pharmacy Peppermint, Tea Tree, Eucalyptus Face Wash

Moisturizers

- Korres Quercetin & Oak Anti-Wrinkle Cream

- Aesop Fabulous Face Oil
- Jurlique Herbal Recovery Night Cream
- Egyptian Magic
- Intelligent Nutrients Certified Organic Anti-Aging Moisture
- Kate Somerville Oil-Free Moisturizer
- Belli Healthy Glow Facial Hydrator

Eye Cream

- Belli Eye Brightening Cream
- Yes to Blueberries Eye Firming Treatment
- Weleda Wild Rose Smoothing Eye Cream
- Naturopathica Primrose Eye and Upper Lip Cream
- REN Active 7 Radiant Eye Maintenance Gel
- ShiKai Borage Dry Skin Therapy Eye Cream

Sunblock

- Belli Anti-Chloasma Facial Sunscreen
- Josie Maran Protect Daily Sun Protection SPF 40
- Super by Perricone Daylight Savings SPF 25 Moisturizer

Lip Care

- Intelligent Nutrients Lip Delivery Nutrition
- EOS Lip Sphere
- Hurraw Moon Balm
- Weleda Everon Lip Balm
- ChapStick 100% Naturals Lip Butter

We also love using the lanolin balms that are traditionally used for nursing discomfort as a treatment for dry, chapped lips. Lanolin instantly soothes and adds a natural glossy sheen to the lips.

Acne Treatment

- Belli Acne Control Spot Treatment

Ever hear the phrase "happy mother, happy baby"? Well, we fully subscribe to that theory. In fact, some studies have linked maternal stress to behavioral problems in their children. There is no reason why any mom-to-be has to go around stressed-out about acne or other skin conditions or feel unattractive during pregnancy. Again, it's just about making those smart choices, which can work in reverse too: making smarter choices actually makes you feel more beautiful. And thanks to people like Josie Maran, there are some amazing products out there that are both smart *and* effective.

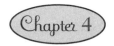

Chapter 4

Mom-Smart Body and Hair Care

The average woman will shower and wash her hair every day during her pregnancy—that's 270 times over nine months. And if you're like us, you wash your hands each day more times than you can remember. As simple as we like to keep things during pregnancy, we'd never suggest dropping toothpaste, shampoo, soap, or deodorant from your routine. In fact, maintaining dental hygiene and keeping your hands clean are two of the most important personal care rituals during pregnancy. But just think about how easily and how often the questionable ingredients in some of these common personal care products could sneak into your daily routine. We dug deep to find the safest, most practical ways to keep your body smelling good, your teeth sparkling, and your hair shiny without compromising on safety.

Brush Up on Dental Care

"Oral health equals overall health," says renowned New York City dentist Dr. Jonathan Levine. "The gums are much more susceptible to plaque during pregnancy because of all the hormonal changes."

Translation? Moms-to-be need to see their dentist more often. If you normally go to the dentist every six months, you should go every three to four months. That's probably not what you want to hear, but prevention is key when it comes to a safe pregnancy. When your teeth are not cared for properly through daily brushing and flossing as well as professional cleaning, plaque—a sticky film composed of bacteria, mucus, and food debris—can build up and produce toxins that may irritate your gums and lead to gingivitis (aka gum or periodontal disease).

Now here's the scary part about gum disease. According to a five-year study conducted at the University of North Carolina at Chapel Hill, pregnant women with moderate to severe gum disease may be seven times more likely to go into preterm labor or to deliver low-birth-weight babies than women with healthy gums.[1] Research suggests that the bacteria in the gums can release toxins into the bloodstream that reach the placenta and interfere with fetal development. The infection can also stimulate a woman's body to produce chemicals that cause the cervix to dilate and set off uterine contractions. Premature birth is not only the major cause of newborn death but also places a baby at greater risk of developing serious and long-term health complications. So if there is ever a time to become vigilant about your oral care, it's during pregnancy.

The good news is that using an alcohol-free mouthwash during pregnancy—especially if you have gingivitis—can greatly reduce the risk of preterm labor or delivering a low-birth-weight baby. A recent study out of the University of Pennsylvania School of Dental Medicine gathered a group of seventy-one pregnant women who had been diagnosed with gingivitis. The group was separated into two subgroups, one of which was told to rinse their mouths twice daily for thirty seconds with an over-the-counter, alcohol-free mouthwash containing cetylpyridinium chloride (CPC), while the other group rinsed only with water. The researchers checked in with the women throughout their pregnancies and found that the risk of preterm delivery among the women who used the mouthwash was reduced by a whopping 75 percent.[2] So pregnancy is an excellent time to use mouthwash religiously.

The White Stuff

Whitening your teeth during pregnancy may seem like a good—and innocuous—way to give your look a boost, but exercise caution when using peroxide. Hydrogen peroxide is a natural substance made up of hydrogen and oxygen molecules. It is a strong oxidizing agent that has a bleaching effect on teeth, hair, skin, and bone. "From the 6 percent [peroxide] consumer whiteners all the way to the professional formulas, which are 20 percent [peroxide], I would say to wait until after the baby comes to do a whitening procedure with the peroxide gel," says Dr. Levine. His advice is to use a good toothbrush like a Sonicare, floss well, keep the gums healthy, and err on the safe side. If you're looking for a safer way to whiten your teeth, try eating apples. Rich in malic acid, which has a natural bleaching effect, apples are also low in calories, and they taste great too!

Healthy Food = Healthy Teeth

Your baby's first teeth start to develop sometime around the end of the first trimester. Eating a healthy diet with a lot of calcium is good for your baby's developing teeth, gums, and bones. If you are looking for ways to add calcium to your diet other than just gulping down the obvious—milk, yogurt, cheese, and Ben & Jerry's—here's our favorite calcium-rich foods:

- Kale (we love kale roasted in the oven with a little salt and olive oil)

- Almonds (one of our favorite lunch sandwiches is almond butter and jelly!)
- Chickpeas and tahini paste (in other words—hummus!)
- Rice pudding (a great way to justify having dessert)
- Salmon (a pregnancy-smart fish because it registers low on the mercury scale)
- Sardines (cut down on the briny taste by tossing them into a pasta dish)

It turns out that healthy eating isn't just good for your growing baby—it's also beneficial to your teeth. "The best thing is eating properly. Nutrition is so critical," says Dr. Levine. "Take it easy on the sweets and the sticky foods. Load up on the fruits and veggies; they're good exfoliants and naturally remove the stains off the teeth."

Dr. Levine's Favorite Pregnancy-Smart Products

- Sonicare toothbrush ("It goes off every thirty seconds to remind you to move to the next area.")
- Dental floss ("Only 10 percent of the population flosses regularly. Pregnancy is a great time to establish a good flossing habit.")
- Arm & Hammer toothpaste with baking soda ("Use a natural toothpaste with no saccharine, no sodium lauryl sulfate [SLS], and low-level fluoride.")
- Sugar-free gum ("Sugar-free gum is great—it increases the saliva, and saliva is a buffering agent.")

Need to Know

Toothbrushes are sponges for bacteria. Let your toothbrush air-dry and replace it every forty-five days.

Hair Care

Pregnancy has a radical effect on the body, and your hair is no exception. Normally, the hairs on your head are in one of three phases: growing, resting, or falling out (mostly when we brush or wash our hair) before the whole process gets repeated. During pregnancy more of the hairs enter the resting phase, and many women experience thicker hair, which is a nice little beauty boost. This is such an important time to care for your hair, not only because there's more of it, but also because having more good hair days can make you feel prettier during a time when your body is getting bigger and bigger. Three to four months after pregnancy, those resting hairs will move on to the falling-out phase, and then the cycle will return to normal.

As a mom-to-be, making sure your hair products aren't rife with potentially harmful ingredients is more important than doing whatever it takes to have shiny and bouncy hair. Shampoo stays on your scalp for a short period of time before it's rinsed off, so you may think it's not that big of a deal, but conditioners can stay in your hair all day. Just remember—the scalp is not a barrier, so proceed with caution. Hair follicles are a natural entry point for chemicals into the skin, and there are about 100,000 of them on your head. How much do the follicles let in? In one study, topical caffeine was absorbed into skin ten times faster when the hair follicles were intact than when they were blocked—and caffeine was detected in the bloodstream almost immediately.[3]

Shampoos use surfactants to clean away dirt and oil. These are chemicals with a special structure that lets them mix with either water or oil. Surfactants also like to stick to themselves; lathering foam and bubbles is what you see when you rub them together and air is trapped inside the mixture. Some surfactants contain sulfates, and while the sulfates themselves can be harsh to the hair, research shows that it's sodium lauryl sulfate that is linked to birth defects, not sodium laureth sulfate. Both sodium lauryl sulfate and sodium laureth sulfate are very common shampoo ingredients. Here's what Dr. Rubin has to say on the subtle but important difference between them: "The FDA, the TGA [Therapeutic Goods Administration], the American Cancer Society, and the Cosmetic, Toiletry, and Fragrance Association all agree that sodium laureth sulfate is safe to use in cosmetic formulations. The ingredient also passes teratology screening cleanly, which means that it has never been linked to birth defects or other problems with pregnancy in published medical research studies."

Many of the ingredients to avoid in your shampoos and conditioners are the same ones you are trying to avoid in your body washes and lotions, such as parabens, retinyl palmitate, aloe, calendula (a potent source of vitamin A) and phthalates (think about how many shampoos and conditioners have fragrances—a lot!). One of our favorite shampoos uses rosemary as a key ingredient, but since rosemary has been linked to reduced fertility in animal studies, we cut that out during pregnancy.

Another popular personal care ingredient that has been in the news recently is methylisothiazolinone (MIT), a commonly used preservative in shampoos and conditioners. Research conducted at the University of Pittsburgh in 2006 showed that MIT inhibits the growth of immature nerve cells in rats in a test tube.[4] Again, since it's unethical to do testing on pregnant women, it's hard to say what effect MIT has on people, but if the University of Pittsburgh research results later turn out to be applicable to living organisms, then it could be that MIT causes neurodevelopmental problems in the developing fetus after mom is exposed. Using products with MIT in them is not a risk we feel is worth taking.

Why I Cut Down on the "Poo": A Note from Melissa

Have you heard about the underground beauty revolution under way? People are saying no to "poo"—shampoo, that is. A very famous hair-stylist to the stars (who has gorgeous hair himself) admits that he never washes his hair with shampoo. He's not the only one to swear by the no-poo approach. A lot of people are throwing in the towel on shampoo and loving the transformation to shiny, bouncy locks. They're not forgoing the shower or water, but just cutting out the shampoo and going straight to the conditioner. Many people who try this method aren't so happy with the results at first, but then begin to see a marked improvement in their hair after a few weeks. Dry, frizzy hair becomes soft and silky.

I think there's no better time to give the no-poo method a shot than during pregnancy. One less product means fewer chemicals to be concerned about. Here's why no-poo converts are giving up the bottle for good. The scalp produces natural oils that give the hair shine and protect it against damage. The more you wash your hair, the more your body produces these oils, leading to the greasy hair that you feel "needs" to be washed every day. Not only that, but the harsh chemicals in some shampoos actually damage the hair. Most no-poo types say that their hair got worse before it got better after they gave up the shampoo. So stick with it for a few weeks before you decide to get back on the poo.

There's also a middle way: My routine of washing my hair only once a week, at most, really keeps my hair from getting dry and frizzy.

The Big Brush-Off

What if we told you that the breakage and dryness your hair experiences during pregnancy and afterward could be helped just by the simple act of brushing your hair? Well, it can.

During pregnancy, your hair grows faster, thanks to all of the estrogen surging through your body, so you have all the more reason to care for it properly, and brushing is one of the best—and easiest—ways to do so. "The greatest beauty secret is not an old wives' tale," says celebrity hair guru Eva Scrivo. "Brushing your hair not only removes dead skin cells at the scalp, but it brings the natural hair oils down the hair shaft." She advises brushing with either a pure boar bristle brush, if you have finer hair, or a boar and plastic blend brush for thicker hair. "It will be more effective than any synthetic conditioner because you're using your own natural oils. It's the most holistic beauty secret out there—simple hair brushing," she says.

Beauty insiders (including us and Scrivo) love the brushes from Mason Pearson, an English company that's been around since the 1800s. These brushes are an investment, as most models are over $100, but it's truly one worth making. "Think of all the products we buy hoping for a miracle when most of the damage could have been eliminated by simple hair brushing," says Scrivo, who also likes using ayurvedic oils in conjunction with brushing. She uses Neem Oil, which is incredibly healing, conditioning, and antiseptic. Want another benefit of brushing? If you're not so keen on washing your hair every day, brushing your hair is another way to clean it: regular brushing lifts away dirt and pollution, so you don't have to wash your hair as often.

What You Should Know About Hair Spray

The occasional use of small amounts of hair spray in a well-ventilated area is considered nontoxic. However, exposure to large amounts of hair spray is another story. A condition called "hair spray poisoning" can result from directly inhaling large amounts of hair spray. Symptoms range from eye and throat burning and skin rash to breathing difficulty to coma, depending on the amount of exposure.

In one human pregnancy study, mothers who reported using hair sprays frequently at work were found to have male infants with an increased risk of hypospadias—a birth defect in which the urethra, the hole in the tip of the penis, opens abnormally along the underside of the penis.[5] The authors of this study speculated that phthalates in the hair spray were responsible for the effect, but since they did not study the ingredients individually, they couldn't determine the exact cause.

Phthalates are hormone-disrupting chemicals that are added to many cosmetics, perfumes, and personal care products as part of a synthetic fragrance mixture. It's difficult to guard against them because they don't show up on the ingredients list. Manufacturers only have to list the word "fragrance"—they don't have to tell you which chemicals are included in the "fragrance." One of your options is to look for products that contain no fragrance. Another is to look for products that claim to be "fragrance-free" or "phthalate-free." If you're still not sure about a product, try contacting the manufacturer to ask whether it includes phthalates.

Kitchen Confidential

Pregnancy hair can look frizzy and dull and be prone to breakage. Make your own yogurt hair mask by whisking one egg until frothy. Then blend in half a cup of plain yogurt and two tablespoons of olive oil. Apply to damp hair in sections. Leave on for at least fifteen minutes, then shampoo and condition as usual. The lactic acid in the yogurt will smooth and hydrate your strands.

Hair Today, Gone Tomorrow

If you're noticing more than just the usual errant dark hair on your face, you can thank your surging hormones for that. Hormonal changes during pregnancy are the culprit for many things, and unfortunately an increase in facial hair is one of them. So what can be done to remove facial hair in a way that's safe and as pain-free as possible? (Remember, when you're pregnant, your skin is ultra-sensitive.) Here's a breakdown of your hair-removing options and just how smart they are:

- *Waxing:* Here's where the sensitivity issue comes into play. Waxing won't harm your fetus, but it will certainly take a toll on your tender upper lip. So proceed with caution. Your skin may not react the same way it did before you got pregnant.
- *Bleaching:* This product stays on the surface of the skin for at least a few minutes during the lightening process, and that may be enough time to start entering the bloodstream. Not to mention the nasty odor. Just say no to bleaching while pregs.
- *Threading:* In this ancient method, a cotton thread works as a lasso, pulling unwanted hairs out of the follicle. Since no chemicals are used in this process, it's completely safe during pregnancy and nursing. Another huge plus is the speed factor. A whole face can be done in just a few minutes. We give this method two thumbs up!
- *Plucking:* This old-school method definitely gets our vote for the safest, but also the most painful. If you can stand yanking one hair out at a time, then go for it. Try numbing the area with ice first and use an angled, sharp-tipped tweezer.
- *Laser hair removal:* This one falls in the "wait until after baby arrives" category. "Laser therapy is contraindicated during

pregnancy because of the risk of hyperpigmentation," says Dr. Alexiades-Armenakas. "The elevated levels of hormones increase the risk of developing pigment wherever your skin is traumatized or lasered. The other risk is, it's really bad for pain and discomfort, and so that presents a risk to the fetus." See the sidebar in Chapter 6 about the effects of stress during pregnancy on children.

Body Care

Keep It Clean: Soaps

One of the first products we looked into is probably the most used product in our health and hygiene regimen, and for good reason—soap. Soap gets things clean in many ways and has no standard active ingredient. It's an emulsification agent that, in conjunction with warm water, binds to dirt and germs and rinses them off the skin. According to the Centers for Disease Control and Prevention (CDC), proper hand washing is one of the most important ways to avoid getting sick. (The average human hand has anywhere from ten thousand to ten million bacteria sitting on the surface!) And if there's one thing you don't want to be while pregnant it's sick.

For soaps, we prefer ingredients like olive oil, sodium chloride, sodium coco-sulfate, beeswax, and vegetable glycerin over triclosan, chloroxylenol (PCMX), triclocarban, BHT, and tetrasodium EDTA. The preservative BHT has been found to cause the congenital absence of one or both eyes in animal studies. Triclosan, which prevents bacterial contamination and is used in many antibacterial soaps, is a suspected toxicant. It creates dioxin, a known carcinogen, as a by-product. The Food and Drug Administration stated in 2010 that "valid concerns" have been raised about triclosan's safety and possible effects on our health. According to the FDA, triclosan alters hormone regulation in animal studies.[6] A study at the University of California at Davis found that triclocarban can alter hormonal activity in rats and in human cells in the laboratory.[7] One million pounds of triclosan and triclocarban are used annually, while triclosan is found in the urine of 75 percent of the population! Chloroxylenol is also a suspected immunotoxin and skin or sense organ toxicant, as well as a gastrointestinal and liver toxicant.

The FDA states on its website that it is "reviewing all of the available evidence on [triclosan's] safety in consumer products and will communicate the findings of its review to the public in winter 2012." As a pregnant woman, you have no reason to wait until then to find out whether this ingredient is safe or not. You can decide now not to mess around with hormone regulation, especially at such a vulnerable time for your growing baby. Hormones are central to regulating fetal growth and critical for proper development of everything from the brain to the lungs to the liver.

Tetrasodium EDTA is a preservative and stabilizer derived from the carcinogenic ingredients formaldehyde and sodium cyanide. As a penetration enhancer, it breaks down the skin's protective barrier and makes it easier for a product to enter the bloodstream, something you definitely want to avoid during pregnancy. Many companies trying to manufacture healthy products use tetrasodium EDTA in place of parabens as a preservative, but beware: it might be just as harmful.

What's more, research has shown that soaps containing these antibacterial chemicals are no more effective than soaps without them. At the University of Wisconsin at La Crosse, a comparative study was done among three soaps: a liquid (non-antibacterial) soap, a chloroxylenol antibacterial soap, and a more common triclosan antibacterial soap. They found that all three soaps effectively reduced the amount of bacteria found on hands and that there was no difference in their effectiveness. The researchers concluded that it's actually the act of vigorously rubbing soap and water on the hands for at least ten seconds that gets rid of bacteria.[8]

Even though good old-fashioned hand washing is our preferred method of cleaning, we carry alcohol-free hand sanitizers with us everywhere. Alcohol is not our favorite ingredient for a whole host of reasons. BabyGanics founder Kevin Schwartz sums it up: "In order for an alcohol-based antibacterial gel to have the appropriate kill claims to be on market, it has to have more than 62 percent alcohol by content. Vodka is 40 percent. This is why you hear about prisoners drinking alcohol-based hand sanitizers." You've probably heard that excessive alcohol intake causes a group of birth defects known as "fetal alcohol syndrome." Though we try to avoid anything with links to birth defects, scientists have studied alcohol consumption very carefully in relation to human pregnancies, and it seems unlikely that your skin would absorb enough to put you at risk. Alcohol is used in topical hand sanitizers because of its germ-killing properties and the fact that it's super-fast-drying. "There are two issues with that," explains Schwartz. "The first issue is that the second it dries off it no longer has any germ-fighting properties, so a minute later, if there's some sort of germ or bacteria that enters the area, you need to sanitize again. The other issue is that it dries out the skin and causes an incredible amount of irritation and dry, cracked skin." Cracked skin due to extreme dryness can lead to increased topical absorption of other ingredients, so beware.

Why Some Deodorants Are the Pits

Google the words "deodorant" and "cancer," and you're likely to scare yourself into tossing all your underarm products in the trash immediately. The reports link aluminum-based compounds, the active ingredients found in most deodorants and antiperspirants, to breast cancer. Here's what the National Cancer Institute (NCI) has to say about the link: "Some research suggests that aluminum-based compounds, which are applied frequently and left on the skin near the breast, may be absorbed by the skin and cause *estrogen*-like (hormonal) effects. Because estrogen has the ability to promote the growth of breast cancer *cells,* some scientists have suggested that the aluminum-based compounds in antiperspirants may contribute to the development of breast cancer. Some research has focused on parabens, which are preservatives used in some deodorants and antiperspirants that have been shown to mimic the activity of estrogen in the body's cells."

The NCI researchers go on to say: "Because studies of antiperspirants and deodorants and breast cancer have provided conflicting results, additional research is needed to investigate this relationship and other factors that may be involved."

Besides their possible links to cancer, some paraben preservatives that were once commonly used in antiperspirants and deodorants (like butylparaben and propylparaben) are also linked to birth defects in published studies. Although it would be better to just avoid parabens altogether, they are used so often in cosmetic products that we know that might be difficult. If you can't find a paraben-free product, look for one that uses only methylparaben—this paraben has less estrogenic potential, and there is no specific evidence that it is harmful during pregnancy.

Other common deodorant and antiperspirant ingredients linked to birth defects or developmental and reproductive problems are aloe, PEG 20, propylene glycol, triclosan, sodium benzoate, and trisodium EDTA. Some of these are the same troublesome ingredients found in soap. Aloe, which acts as an anti-irritant, is typically considered safe, but during pregnancy it has been linked to an increased rate of embryonic deaths in animal studies. The same is true of propylene glycol, which is used in some products to give them "slip" (to prevent the escape of moisture or water). And PEG 20 may contain harmful impurities, such as 1,4-dioxane, which is a known carcinogen.

Because these questionable ingredients are found in almost all the standard deodorants on the market, we are left with a dearth of good odor-maskers. The problem is that finding a deodorant that not only has healthy ingredients but actually works is Holy Grail territory. We spritzed, sprayed, and rolled pretty much every "natural" brand of deodorant under the sun and were still left smelling pitty. However, we did find a few products that not only masked our smelliness but also looked to be safer than many others on the market.

"I didn't want to use a crystal or a wipe and was so tired of not finding a natural alternative that was effective," concurs Lavanila cofounder Danielle Raynor, maker of one of our favorite pregnancy-smart deodorants. "It took us about two years of research and development to create this proprietary technology that uses beta glucan to feed the skin as opposed to clogging the pores. It actually nourishes the skin without the use of aluminum or parabens."

Fragrance and Pregnancy

One of the most synthetically produced products you can put on your skin is fragrance. Some fragrances contain hundreds of unlisted ingredients, including many phthalates, which as we know has links to birth defects. Fragrance is not limited to perfume. You may not realize that fragrance is also found in most of your personal care products to mask the odor of the other chemicals in the mix. If you look at the ingredients of your scented beauty products, you will most likely see "fragrance" or "parfum" listed on the back. But when you're spritzing that bottle of perfume or applying a cream or lotion with "parfum" or "fragrance" as one of its ingredients, it's impossible to know what chemicals you're exposing yourself to—and your baby.

Because fragrance formulas are considered trade secrets, US manufacturers are not required to list the ingredients. However, if the Safe Cosmetics Act of 2011, which was introduced on Capitol Hill in June 2011, is passed by Congress, that will change. One of the act's provisions is a requirement that manufacturers list the ingredients in a fragrance. Other provisions include mandatory reporting of adverse health effects by the manufacturer. (Go to safecosmetics.org for more information.)

Melissa gets an instant headache when she walks through the perfume floor of a major department store. Many people have the same sensitivity to fragrance. From sneezing to watery eyes to nausea and skin rashes, there are whole host of reactions provoked by fragrance. According to the American Academy of Dermatology, exposure to fragrance in skincare products is a main cause of skin allergies. It does help to know that responsible skincare companies will do RIPT (repeat insult patch testing) to allergy test their products and will not market them if adverse reactions were seen on the test subjects.

The olfactory assault of fragrance is a lot like second hand smoke exposure. A fragranced product affects everyone who breathes it in, not just the person wearing it. A study conducted by a group of researchers, including Lance A. Wallace from the Environmental Protection Agency (EPA), found 133 different volatile organic compounds (VOCs) emitted from the 25 common fragranced consumer products they investigated, with an average of 17 VOCs per product. Of these 133 VOCs, 24 were classified as toxic or hazardous under US federal laws, and each product emitted at least one of these compounds.[9] According to the EPA: "VOCs are emitted as gases from certain solids or liquids. VOCs include a variety of chemicals, some of which may have short- and long-term adverse health effects."

Let's not forget that pregnancy makes you super sensitive to smells. So even if there's a perfume you've always loved, it may be a trigger for a migraine or nausea while you're pregnant. It's kind of amazing how Mother Nature knows what moms-to-be should avoid. Drinking caffeine and alcohol can also trigger nausea during pregnancy—more evidence that your body knows what's best to avoid.

The best approach is to try and cut out every product with synthetic fragrances during pregnancy. This not only protects your fetus from the chemicals in the fragrance, it also helps protect you from being struck with an awful migraine or a sudden need to toss your cookies.

If you really love your perfume and don't think you can go all nine months without it, then we advise at least cutting it out for the first trimester. A recent study proposed a possible link between perfume usage during the first twelve weeks of pregnancy and problems with reproductive systems. According to the study, male rats born to mothers who were exposed to perfume during the first twelve weeks of pregnancy were more apt to suffer from infertility or undescended testes. The reasoning is that the chemicals in perfume may block androgen release, which is crucial for the development of the male reproductive system.

The beauty vets behind Lavanila were sick of spraying synthetic chemicals onto their skin too. Lavanila fragrances are free of synthetic chemicals and instead packed with antioxidants. Another option for smelling good is the use of essential oils, which have the added benefit of lifting your mood. Research shows that some natural fragrances can act as antidepressants. There was a study conducted at the Mie University School of Medicine in Japan that showed citrus fragrance to have an antidepressant effect. When given to twelve different people suffering depression, the scent of citrus helped so much that the results indicated that the doses of antidepressant medication could be reduced.[10]

Even though, for now, you won't see the ingredients listed on the back of your perfume packages, here are some common fragrance chemicals linked to birth defects: methylene chloride, toluene, methyl ethyl ketone, methyl isobutyl ketone, tert butyl, sec butyl, and benzyl chloride.[11]

Mama Says

I stopped using perfume when I was breast-feeding. I switched to jojoba oil—it's less expensive and a lot safer. I also cut out a lot of home cleaning products when my daughter was born. I bought a steam cleaner and cleaned my house mostly with vinegar, baking soda, and steam.

—MARY BRUNE,
cofounder of MOMS (Making Our Milk Safe)

Pregnancy Body Issues

Some women, bless them, claim to feel their most beautiful during pregnancy. It's hard to deny that overall feeling of excitement and purpose with a growing life inside you. But neither of us felt as though we were at our beauty peak during pregnancy. Melissa dealt with majorly swollen (and painful!) breasts, while Annette battled edema in her legs and feet and a tendency to form stretch marks. Sometimes you have to just throw in the towel and let your body do what it's got to do, but we do have some strategies to make pregnancy body issues a little easier to bear. Here's how to deal with some of the most common complaints.

Common Scents: A Note from Annette

It's no secret that pregnancy makes us aroma-sensitive. When creating the Belli pregnancy collection, we asked women what they wanted to smell like during pregnancy, and they said, "Fresh and clean." I was uncertain whether "fresh and clean" meant Ivory soap, cucumber kiwi, or coconut vanilla. So I arranged a focus group with pregnant mamas to get a better understanding of what exactly "fresh and clean" meant. The citrus family won, with lemon at the top of the list. Peppermint and lavender also scored high as appealing scents. The aromatherapy of peppermint and lemon is believed to ease morning sickness and upset stomach.

Stretch Marks

During the second and third trimesters, your uterus will grow rapidly, stretching the skin over your abdomen and tearing the connective tissues in the dermis. Sounds lovely, huh? The torn tissue heals with irregular scars, also known as stretch marks (*Striae gravidarum*). The growth of fat deposits in the breasts, hips, thighs, and buttocks can cause stretch marks in these areas as well. Stretch marks affect 70 to 90 percent of all women. They occur more often in first pregnancies, the fair-skinned, and the overweight. There is definitely a genetic component, so you may not be able to avoid them, but you can minimize your risk by avoiding excessive weight gain and staying well hydrated.

So what ingredients can you rely on to help avoid stretch marks? Although generations of moms-to-be have used cocoa butter to try to prevent stretch marks, a recent study shows no benefits at all from this ingredient (although it's a good moisturizer).[12] However, there was one study that showed that a combination of several topical ingredients (including gotu kola and vitamin E) decreases the risk of stretch marks by about 39 percent and decreases the severity of any stretch marks that do form.[13]

Annette's Belli Beautiful Prescription for Stretch Marks

Isn't it interesting that as soon as we are expecting we begin to really appreciate our former bodies? Our pre-pregnancy figure all of a sudden doesn't seem so imperfect, and our desire to preserve it becomes almost an obsession for some of us. The most common pregnancy skin care concerns that women voice are: (1) is there anything out there that can prevent stretch marks? and (2) what do I do if I already have them? We've already established that there is no magic potion that you can rub on your stomach that comes with a 100 percent guarantee it will prevent stretch marks. But research points to several promising ingredients—like gotu kola and vitamin E (tocopherol)—that, combined with other beauty-boosters, are found in Belli's Elasticity Belly Oil.

During my pregnancy, I added some skin-saving rituals to my daily routine that would help prepare my skin for stretching. My routine looked like this:

1. I massaged Belli's Fresh Start Pre-Treatment Scrub into areas where I had concerns about getting stretch marks. I used the scrub four to five times weekly on lightly dampened skin, but if you're not a veteran of exfoliation, try gradually working your way up to an every-other-day scrub-down.
2. I would then get out of the shower, towel off, and massage Elasticity Belly Oil over my freshly exfoliated skin. In no more than a minute, my body would feel like I had just been to my favorite five-star spa.

Now let's shift gears and talk about minimizing the appearance of the stretch marks we already have. Most of us get stretch marks during pregnancy, but they can also happen during the growth spurts of puberty or from rapid weight loss or weight gain. Stretch marks fade naturally to some extent, but they never go away completely. Dozens of cosmetic products claim to help fade stretch marks. Some of them even have great research behind them. When we looked at all the evidence, we found two ingredients that seemed particularly effective. Darutoside, from the plant *Siegesbeckia orientalis,* was shown in scientific research to reduce the appearance of a stretch mark's length and irregular surface area by up to 52 percent, and registril, derived from green beans, reduces the appearance of a stretch mark's depth by up to 72 percent.[14]

Here's my recommended regimen to restore your skin after pregnancy:

- In the shower, exfoliate over the stretch marks every other day.
- Towel-dry and then apply your stretch mark product to the affected areas twice daily. Massaging the area is also thought to be helpful in reducing the appearance of these marks—so try massaging while exfoliating or applying any other body product.
- Ask your dermatologist about prescription solutions, such as retinoids or laser treatments.

Swelling and Water Retention

If you're having trouble sliding on your wedding ring or getting into your favorite pair of shoes, don't worry, you're not the only one. Women retain 30 percent more water in the bloodstream during pregnancy to help with fetal development. Gravity forces some of this water out of the blood vessels and into the tissues of the legs and feet, where it causes painful swelling known as *peripheral edema*.

This condition tends to be worse after a long day of standing or walking. It is also worse in the third trimester, when the growing uterus pushes on the largest vein in the body (the *vena cava*), which further raises the pressure of the water being pushed out into the tissues.

There are no topical ingredients or products that can reduce pregnancy-related swelling. Mild swelling is best relieved by taking short breaks during the day to lie down and elevate your legs above the level of your heart. Light massage of the swollen areas helps relieve swelling and feels great too. Swelling that is persistent or severe, however, or that involves the face and hands may be an early sign of pre-eclampsia—a potentially dangerous condition. See your physician immediately if you experience this kind of swelling.

Dry, Itchy Skin

We both had a bad case of the itches on our tummies during our pregnancies. Melissa even had the unfortunate experience of developing an allergic reaction, which led to red, itchy hives all over her body. That degree of itchiness is rare, but many women experience dry skin at some point during their pregnancy. Itching is more common over tightly stretched areas of skin, such as the abdomen, in the second and third trimesters. Another cause of itching is cholestasis, a condition in which slower liver function loads the skin with bile salts. Some women even develop jaundice and gallstones. Other causes of itching include drug reaction, atopic dermatitis, and contact allergies. Finally, although there are many other kinds of rashes during pregnancy, most of them, fortunately, are rare.

Consult with a dermatologist for itching that is persistent, severe, or associated with red bumps or blisters on the skin. We found that the best way to treat dry, itchy skin is to moisturize morning, noon, and night. Keep a bottle of (pregnancy-friendly) lotion at your desk and in the bathroom. Both showering and washing your hands can lead to excessive dryness, so be sure to apply your moisturizer as soon as you dry off.

Varicose and Spider Veins

When you're pregnant, your body produces extra blood to support you and your growing baby—about 50 percent more, in fact. This increased amount of blood fills your veins to capacity. Your enlarging uterus pushes against the vena cava, which increases the pressure in the veins of your pelvis and legs. As you stand throughout the day, gravity puts even more pressure on those veins. All of these factors contribute to an increased risk of getting varicose veins or spider veins.

Varicose veins are enlarged, superficial veins that appear swollen and bulging above the surface of the skin. They can be blue, red, purplish, or flesh-colored and usually appear on the lower half of the body. Spider veins are like varicose veins but smaller and more spread out. They are also closer to the surface of the skin and may be found on any area of the body—though they are most frequently seen on the legs and face. They appear reddish or bluish in color and look like small spiderwebs—hence the name.

Here's how you can help prevent and lessen the severity of varicose and spider veins:

* Keep moving! Daily exercise that increases circulation is one of the best ways to prevent varicose veins. As your muscles expand and contract, they push your blood up through your veins and help prevent the blood from pooling.

- When sitting down, try to keep your legs elevated and avoid sitting with your legs crossed. Propping your feet up above the level of your heart helps to counteract the effect of gravity on the veins. Crossed legs can compress the veins even more, so do your best to help that blood move along!
- Avoid gaining extra weight. Carrying unnecessary pounds increases the demands on your already stressed circulatory system. The optimal weight gain for average-sized women is twenty-five to thirty-five pounds.
- Sleep on your left side so as to move the uterus off of the vena cava and help to maximize venous blood flow.
- Practice safe sun. Too much sun exposure can raise the risk of spider veins on the face.
- Have your partner massage your lower legs with effleurage movements (long, light strokes), which can encourage circulation and help prevent venous pooling. Promise a back rub in return.
- Steer clear of heavy lifting and straining, which puts an extra burden on your veins and also is not safe for the baby.
- Wear support hosiery. Find an over-the-counter gradient compression hose. They give more support than the traditional support pantyhose. We recommend Preggers by Therafirm for a line of pantyhose, tights, leggings, and trouser socks in a broad range of fashionable colors at reasonable prices. Jobst and Gabriella also make support hosiery that comes highly recommended by health care professionals.

Varicose veins can be uncomfortable and a pesky cosmetic issue during pregnancy, but for most women varicose veins shrink or disappear a few months after you have given birth. There also seems to be a genetic component to varicose veins: if you have them during one pregnancy, there's a good chance they will recur in all of your pregnancies, so be sure to take extra precautions.

Talk to your physician about the best options for handling varicose veins that stick around long after your baby arrives. The most common treatment is sclerotherapy: the doctor injects a liquid chemical directly into the vein that causes it to shrink and wither. Other options include surface laser treatments, endovenous techniques, and surgery.

You should talk to your doctor about your varicose veins if:

- One of the varicose veins begins to bleed
- Your leg symptoms are interfering with regular daily activities
- The varicose vein becomes warm to the touch, red, very tender, or swollen
- You see a rash or sores on your leg or ankle
- The veins become painful

Superficial varicose veins should not be confused with another more serious problem called *deep venous thrombosis*. In this condition, a blood clot starts to form in the larger veins deep inside your leg muscles or up inside your pelvis. The blood clot can grow very large, and the big risk is that a piece of it will break off, flow up through the veins, travel through the right side of the heart, and end up inside the lungs, where it becomes trapped inside the smaller pulmonary arteries and arterioles. The sudden blockage prevents oxygen and other vital nutrients from reaching the delicate lung tissue further downstream, and part of the lung starts to die. This is called a pulmonary embolism, and it can be life-threatening. Pregnant women are at increased risk of developing deep venous thrombosis and pulmonary embolism, so it's important that you know the warning signs.

Talk to your doctor immediately if you have any of the following symptoms:

- Increasing pain, swelling, or redness in the legs
- Sudden onset of a sharp chest pain or shortness of breath

How to Be a Skin-Smart Nursing Mama

We all want our babies to have the healthiest start in life, and it's well-known that breast-feeding is one of the best ways to secure both short- and long-term health benefits for our little ones. The first breast milk (*colostrum*) that your body produces contains large amounts of *secretory immunoglobulin A* (IgA). This substance helps guard against invading germs by forming a protective layer in your baby's intestines, throat, and nose.

As you are exposed to various pathogens, your body responds by making a secretory IgA specific to those pathogens, thus protecting your baby from all those unwanted viruses and bacteria. Along with the immediate boost that breast milk gives to a baby's immune system, studies show, breast-feeding may help children avoid certain diseases later in life, such as acute otitis media (middle ear infections), atopic dermatitis (eczema), obesity, type 1 and 2 diabetes, and (possibly) certain forms of childhood leukemias.[15]

Since we know that some of what we apply topically is absorbed systemically, are there any harmful ingredients we should avoid to ensure that our milk supply is pure and safe? When Belli's physicians asked the same question, they turned to the LactMed database. Part of the National Library of Medicine's

(NLM) Toxicology Data Network (TOXNET), this database of drugs and other chemicals includes information on the levels of substances in breast milk and infant blood and the possible adverse effects in the nursing infant. Here are some of the red-flagged ingredients along with the research showing why they should be avoided during nursing:

Salicylic Acid—the Main Metabolite of Aspirin

- A sixteen-day-old breast-fed infant developed metabolic acidosis with a salicylate serum level of 240 milligrams per liter and salicylate metabolites in the urine. The mother was taking daily aspirin for arthritis.[16]
- Thrombocytopenia, fever, anorexia, and petechiae occurred in a five-month-old breast-fed infant five days after her mother started taking aspirin for fever. One week after recovery, the infant was given a single dose (125 milligrams) of aspirin, and her platelet count dropped once again.[17]
- Hemolysis was seen in a twenty-three-day-old, G-6-PD-deficient, breast-fed infant after the mother took aspirin and phenacetin.[18]

Caffeine

- Jitteriness in a six-week-old breast-fed infant was reported by a mother who claimed to drink four to five cups of coffee and two to three bottles (about 480 milliliters each) of cola daily, as well as occasional tea and cocoa. Upon examination, the infant was gaining weight appropriately, but had trembling and increased muscle tone. The infant's symptoms decreased markedly two weeks after his mother stopped all caffeine-containing beverages.[19]

- Restlessness and irritability were reported in a breast-fed (extent of nursing not stated) five-month-old infant whose mother drank twenty cups of coffee a day.[20]
- A physician who reported drinking at least five mugs of coffee, four mugs of tea, and one can of cola daily breast-fed two infants. The first slept for only brief periods and woke easily. The second baby was fretful and jumpy and also had poor sleep patterns until his mother stopped her caffeine intake.[21]
- Another physician who reportedly drank 1.7 to 2 liters of decaffeinated coffee daily had premature twins (age and extent of nursing not stated) who both seemed to be irritable, although the larger infant was partially supplemented with formula and seemed less affected. When the mother's coffee consumption increased, the smaller infant suffered convulsive-like episodes. All symptoms resolved twenty-four hours after the mother stopped drinking coffee.[22]
- In a study of low-income nursing mothers in Costa Rica, subjects were divided into high-intake coffee drinkers (over 450 milliliters daily) and nondrinkers of coffee. Infants of the coffee drinkers had a lower birth weight and decreased concentrations of maternal and infant hemoglobin and hematocrit at birth. The iron levels in breast milk were also lower among the coffee drinkers, and their infants' hemoglobin and hematocrit values were lower at one month postpartum.[23]

Talcum Powder

You should also try to avoid talcum powder, and use sparingly any products that contain corticoid steroids. Make sure that you avoid using any personal care product directly on your breasts, and gently cleanse them with a clean towel and water before breast-feeding.

The Truth About Nipple Creams

We know that for approximately 30 percent of us, breast-feeding comes with a painful price—sore, dry, cracked, and sometimes bleeding nipples. If you're dealing with this problem, you may be wondering whether there are any products that will comfort and soothe your needy nipples while also meeting our higher safety standards.

The problem here is that, unlike other topical products, nursing creams can be swallowed by newborns in large amounts. With multiple feedings each day, there is a real risk of significant absorption. It's not clear exactly which chemicals are harmful to babies when swallowed in large amounts. A nipple barrier ointment made only from ingredients found in typical baby foods would be fine, but unfortunately, we're not aware of any such product. What we do recommend is the hypoallergenic "medical grade" of lanolin, which has been used for centuries as a nursing cream without any reports of harm or problems, other than allergic reactions. Also, there are no preservative ingredients in lanolin ointments because they are not water-based. Lanolin is also one of those cure-all ingredients that doubles as an amazing lip balm and cuticle cream.

Any ingredients added to a nipple cream run the risk of creating an unpleasant taste or odor that could interfere with your baby's desire to breast-feed. So ask yourself: do I know enough about these ingredients to spoon-feed them straight to my baby? If not, we think it's better to avoid the product. The following are pregnancy-smart nipple creams:

- Lansinoh HPA Lanolin
- Belli Pure Comfort Nursing Cream
- Medela PureLan 100

Mama Says

Your happiness is key to a great, healthy pregnancy—and great, healthy kids. So I think it's really important to check in with yourself every day and ask yourself: am I happy? And if you're not, do what you need to do in order to make yourself happy, because it's all a trickle-down effect. If you're not happy, get out there and take that power walk or run or get a manicure, disappear for half an hour and check in with yourself.

—ELISABETH ROHM, actress

Choose to Use: Mom-Smart Body and Hair Product Picks

Shampoo

- Burt's Bees Super Shiny Grapefruit and Sugar Beet Shampoo
- John Masters Unscented Shampoo
- Prive Concept Vert Shampoo

Conditioner

- Peter Lamas Soy Hydrating Conditioner
- Peter Lamas Avocado and Olive Ultra Smoothing Conditioner
- Know! Conditioner

Body Lotion

- 100 Percent Pure Organic Lavender Nourishing Body Cream
- Eco Tools Replenish Your Natural Resources Body Butter
- California Baby Natural Pregnancy Emulsion
- Terralina Fragrance Free Body Lotion

Deodorant

- Tom's of Maine Long-Lasting Natural Aluminum-Free Deodorant Unscented
- Lavanila: The Healthy Deodorant
- Nature's Gate Herbal Blend Deodorant in Chamomile and Lemon Verbena

Sunblock

- Josie Maran Argan Sun Protection for the Body
- Aubrey Natural Sun SPF 30+

Soap and Body Wash

- Kiss My Face Olive Oil Bar Soap, Pure Olive Oil
- Dove Unscented White Beauty Bar
- Yes To Cucumbers Calming Shower Gel
- Whole Foods Organic Castile Peppermint Soap
- 100 Percent Pure Organic Virgin Coconut Body Wash

Stretch Mark Products

- Erbaviva Stretch Mark Cream
- Belli Elasticity Belly Oil

Hairstyling Products

- Josie Maran Argan Oil Hair Serum
- Couture Colour Pequi Oil Treatment

Hand Sanitizers

- Clean Well Hand Sanitizing Wipes in Orange Vanilla

Changing Your Personal Care Habits

Once we commit to specific brands of products, especially soap, toothpaste, and shampoo, it can be hard to let go of those brands. These products have spent many years with us, and we've used them in the most intimate of places, the bathroom and the shower. We know how hard it is to change brands, but there is no better time to try a new—and safer—brand than during pregnancy. It's especially important for products that you use multiple times a day or apply all over your body. We hope that the products we recommend here will become your new bathroom staples. And trust us: we wouldn't recommend anything that doesn't actually work (especially in the deodorant department!) or that we haven't tried out ourselves.

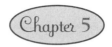
Mom-Smart Makeup

I t's easy to think that topical absorption is not a concern when it comes to color cosmetics since we wash off our makeup every night. But in reality, that's not the case. Considering that, "for many women, their makeup remains on their faces longer than their skin care does"—as Maureen Kelly, founder of Tarte cosmetics and mother of two boys, points out—we should be just as aware of the ingredients in our color cosmetics.

We're hard-core skin care fanatics, but we also believe in the importance of complexion-perfecting makeup. As you know by now, during pregnancy we both took a very conservative approach to skin care. We used only cleanser, moisturizer, eye cream, lip balm, and sun protection. With makeup, we also chose to minimize our product use and go with only the essentials: foundation or tinted moisturizer, concealer where we needed it, a little blush or bronzer, and mascara. On special occasions we broke out the eye shadow, eyeliner, and lip color.

While neither of us felt much like doing a full face of makeup every day (thanks to pregnancy exhaustion), we couldn't face the outside world—or our mirrors—without at least a few secret makeup weapons. We know firsthand the effects of pregnancy fatigue and what that can do to the skin. "When you're tired, you lose pigment in the cheeks," says makeup artist extraordinaire Laura Geller, who learned that when she was pregnant with her son. Later in this chapter, we'll tell you how to transition your makeup routine once you've entered the time-zapping world of motherhood. But first, it's important to understand exactly what ingredients you should be looking for in your color cosmetics during pregnancy.

The Colorful Controversy of Artificial Dyes

The major ingredient difference between makeup and other types of beauty products is color additives. Without them, blush wouldn't make your cheeks rosy, concealer wouldn't conceal, and lipstick wouldn't put any color on your lips. Here's the story behind the sometimes hard-to-understand color ingredients.

When you look at the box of your eyeliner or foundation bottle, you're going to see a lot of letters and numbers, such as FD&C Yellow No. 5, or CI 19140. So what do these codes mean? Color additives in the United States are preapproved by the Food and Drug Administration. After approval, the FDA comes up with the official names for each color additive. Colors subject to batch certification are designated as FD&C (food, drug, and cosmetics), D&C (drug and cosmetics), or Ext. D&C (external drugs and cosmetics). This code is followed by a color designation, such as blue or red, and by a number. Some colors are combined with substrates, such as sodium, potassium, aluminum, barium, calcium strontium, or zirconium. Substrates prevent colors from bleeding, help them to remain stable, and influence the depth of the pigment. These combined colors are known as "lakes." You'll easily be able to decipher these ingredients because they include the word "lake" and the substrate—for example, FD&C Red 40 Lake Aluminum. Our teratology research did not turn up any red flags in relation to any of the commonly used substrates in color cosmetics.

The Color War

When it's time to start feeding your child solid foods, we suggest reading food labels with just as critical an eye as you've brought to your cosmetics. There's been much debate regarding the use of artificial dyes in our food and their possible links to hyperactivity and other behavioral problems in children. In 1975 Dr. Benjamin Feingold wrote a book, called *Why Your Child Is Hyperactive*, in which he posed a link between artificial dyes and hyperactivity (or attention deficit/hyperactivity disorder, ADHD) in kids. Since then, other research has supported that link.[1]

It's easy to understand why artificial coloring is found in makeup, but why is it added to food? Think about it this way: are you more tempted to eat a dull-looking white yogurt or one that's gleaming with bright blueberries and vibrant raspberries? We think you know the answer. There are natural plant- and vegetable-based alternatives to artificial colors, but they are much pricier.

So what happens when those artificial colors are added to the products we use to blush our cheeks, stain our lips, and enhance our eyes? It turns out that artificial dyes (especially the red dyes) are suspected of allergic reaction in a fair number of people. The Environmental Working Group's "Skin Deep" database suggests that, during pregnancy, some dyes—including Acid Yellow 23 Lake Aluminum—may pose development or reproductive risks. Red 30 Lake Aluminum (CI 73360) and Red 28 Lake Aluminum (CI 45410:2) are two other colors called out by the EWG for their links to nervous system birth defects.

While many of the companies that screened clean in our results use the more expensive plant- and vegetable-based colors, it's next to impossible to find a traditional makeup brand that doesn't use artificial color additives. But you should breathe easier knowing that not all of them are thought to be harmful. The dyes that passed our prenatal safety screening include CI 77492 (Iron Oxide Yellow) (Iron Oxides), CI 77491 (Iron Oxides), CI 77499 (Iron Oxides), Manganese Violet (CI 77742), Ultramarine Red, Ultramarine Blue, Red 27 Lake Aluminum (CI 45410), and D&C Red 6 Barium Lake (CI 15850).

The red dyes have been linked more often to allergic reactions, harmful contaminants, and birth defects. For example, in 1976, Red Dye 2 was banned by the FDA because of links to cancer, birth defects, and miscarriage in animals. It's also been reported that trace amounts of lead may lurk in red lipsticks. The matte, longer-lasting, deeply pigmented red lip colors seem to have a higher percentage of lead content. Though some people believe that trace amounts of lead in lipstick carry a low risk of harm, we haven't seen any data that prove this. So we recommend erring on the side of caution during pregnancy and avoiding ruby red lips. Opt instead for lighter-weight gloss versions of your favorites, which generally are more moisturizing and have less pigment in the formulations. Save the red lips for your first post-baby date night, and afterwards break it out only for special occasions.

Seeing Red

And now a little bit about the color that really bugs us. Look on the box of your go-to red lipstick or pink blush and chances are you'll see CI 75470 listed as one of the ingredients. That's the code for carmine, a commonly used dye in food, fabrics, and cosmetics whose color ranges from deep red to magenta. It comes from an insect called a cochineal, a small bug with an impressive past. When Cortés arrived in the New World in 1518, he discovered the use of this dye among the Aztecs. It is said that by the end of the sixteenth century as much as half a million pounds of cochineal was shipped each year from Mexico to Spain, where it was used in lipstick, rouge, and eye makeup. During that time a Spanish galleon sank near Cuba. According to the cargo manifest, the ship contained cochineal with a higher value than New World gold!

Recently the FDA mandated that, starting in 2011, companies using this dye have to list it in the ingredients list as "carmine" after numerous consumer complaints about its allergenic effects. In teratology research, carmine has been cited as the probable cause of rib and vertebral defects in mice.[2] We think it's now time to let the cochineal peacefully inhabit its cactus homes and for us to use more earth- and people-friendly red dye alternatives.

Something to Blink About!

Some mascara formulas contain formaldehyde or the formaldehyde-releasing preservative diazolidinyl urea. This ingredient is a suspected teratogen and should be avoided during pregnancy. During her quest for a replacement, Annette found Zuzu Luxe—an earth-friendly brand of beauty products with a mascara called The Mascara. It delivered as it promised—adding wattage to her wink.

We recommend that during pregnancy you avoid placing the mascara wand at the base of the eyelashes to prevent the product from touching the delicate skin around the eye. (Remember, the eye has mucous membranes, which can absorb chemicals more quickly.) Instead, just coat the tip of your lashes—you'll be surprised by how little product it takes to add a lot of pop.

Another ingredient that is frequently used in mascara, eyeliners, lip pencils, and eye makeup removers is mercury. You've probably been warned by your health care provider to avoid certain types of seafood owing to the high levels of mercury found in them. The World Health Organization explains how the fish became laden with mercury. "Mercury in soaps, creams and other cosmetic products is eventually discharged into wastewater. The mercury enters the environment, where it becomes methylated and enters the food chain as the highly toxic methylmercury in fish. Pregnant women who consume the fish containing the methylmercury transfer the mercury to their fetuses, which can result in neurodevelopmental deficits in the children."[3]

You won't see mercury listed as an ingredient in mascara; look instead for the preservatives phenyl mercuric salts, phenylmercuric acetate, or phenylmercuric nitrate. These are all compounds of mercury; if you see any of them on your ingredient label, toss the product. If you want to take a stand, inform the manufacturer that you won't buy the product as long as these harmful ingredients are used in it. Your voice as a consumer is powerful—use it to make positive changes. Your children and the fish will thank you for it!

Time to Toss?

There's no *good* time to contract a bacterial infection, but pregnancy has got to be the absolute worst time. Some bacteria lurking in makeup can cause serious infections, especially if the product is used on an open cut, like a picked-at zit, or comes into contact with the mucous membranes of the eyes or nose. As a general rule, if you've had any makeup product for longer than a year or it looks or smells weird, toss it in the trash. Using the following list, take an inventory of your collection and determine whether it's time to break up with some of your makeup.

- *Mascara:* The mascara wand loves to attract bacteria before it gets deposited back into the tube. Replace your mascara every two to three months.
- *Eyeliner:* Replace liquid liner about every three months. Just like mascara, liquid liners love to host bacteria. A pencil liner will last much longer, since you're sharpening it and thus removing the area exposed to bacteria. Make sure you keep the lids on your pencils when not in use. Another good habit is to sharpen the pencil frequently to shave off any portion of your pencil that may have been exposed to harmful bacteria. If your eyeliner hardens to the point where it's difficult or even a bit painful to apply, that's a clear sign that the product has dried out because it's old or the cap didn't fit snuggly. Either way, it's time to shop for a new one.
- *Lipstick:* Do not share your lip colors with others, and keep the lid securely on your product to keep it as clean as possible. Although lipstick usually lasts up to two years, if yours starts to smell odd or changes texture, dispose of it and move to a new tube. When sampling lip colors at the cosmetics counter, use the stick part of a cotton swab to gently remove the top and sides of the lip color. Dispose of the color you gently removed and then, with a clean stick, shave a bit of color off and use your fingertip or an unused tester brush to apply the color.
- *Foundation:* Most foundation—save for powder formulations—are packed with water and thus provide a perfect place for bacteria to form. It's important to store your liquid foundations in a cool, dry place and to buy a new one every six to twelve months.
- *Face powder:* Unless it contains water—and most do not—face powder can last a long time. Still, we recommend getting

a new one after one year, especially if you're not diligent about cleaning your makeup brushes.

- *Blush:* Powder blushes can last up to one year if you take care of them. The best way to keep your powder blushes free of ick is to keep your makeup brushes clean. It's recommended that you clean your brushes once a week to rid the bristles of caked-on makeup, oil, and bacteria. Wash them with a mild cleanser and let them dry thoroughly. Regular washing will keep your brushes soft, and your makeup will stay clean and be easier to apply. If you don't clean your brushes often, oil from your face transfers to the brush and then onto your blush. This can cause a layer of film to gather on the surface of your product, making it difficult for your blush brush to "grab" any of the blush.
- *Concealer:* Creamy stick and powder concealers can last up to two years, while liquid ones should be tossed after one year.

Pregnancy Makeup Dos and Don'ts

Do . . .

- Apply mascara to the tips of your lashes only, rather than from the base, where topical absorption can happen.
- Start your makeup routine with a mineral-based sunscreen (see our shopping guide in Chapter 8 for recommended products). The best way to prevent sun damage or chloasma is to use an SPF, and many foundations do not contain adequate SPF.
- Store your makeup in your bedroom or even the fridge instead of the bathroom. Warm, moist areas are great places for breeding bacteria. Go with an area that's cool and dry instead.

Don't...

- Apply makeup on top of broken skin—like concealer on top of a cut or a zit you've just picked at. That's a direct pathway for ingredients to enter the bloodstream.
- Use eyeliner on the inner rims of the eyes during pregnancy. Instead, line only the outer rims. Our favorite place for eyeliner is the top lids, to make eyes look wide awake.
- Share makeup with anyone else while you're pregnant. Personally, we're not fans of ever letting anyone else borrow our mascara, but pregnancy is the time you just want to say no.

Choose to Use: Pregnancy-Smart Makeup Picks

When it came to screening makeup, we had a hard time finding products that stood up to our strict standards. Many skin care companies have come a long way by making their formulations safer, but a lot of our favorite brands of color cosmetics still contain parabens and other not very baby-friendly ingredients. We screened makeup from all over the retail spectrum—from the drugstore to the department store—and found only a handful of brands that we feel it is safe to recommend. That's why you'll see a lot of the same brands repeated in our product picks. That said, we were psyched to discover a lot of these companies during the writing of this book. Not only are their formulations cleaner than the rest, but their products also impressed us.

Tinted Moisturizer

Tip: For a bronzing effect, buy tinted moisturizer a shade darker than your natural skin tone.

- Living Nature Tinted Moisturizer

Foundation

Tip: Always apply your foundation starting at the center of your face. Use your fingers or a makeup sponge or brush (try the Beauty Blender or Tarte's Airbrush Finish Bamboo Foundation Brush) to blend it out gradually around the entire face. What you don't want is that awful line of foundation that stops at your jawbone!

- bareMinerals SPF 15 Foundation
- Maybelline Mineral Power Powder Foundation
- Alima Pure Satin Matte Foundation
- Vapour Atmosphere Luminous Foundation
- Jane Iredale Amazing Base SPF 20
- W3LL Narcissist Stick Foundation
- Dr.Hauschka Translucent Makeup
- NIKA Mineral Makeup
- Living Nature Illuminating Tint

Concealer

Tip: The best way to make dark circles disappear? Look in the mirror closely and you'll see dark pockets in the inner corners of your eyes— those are the areas you want to cover with concealer. The last place you want concealer is on the outer corners of the eyes—you know, where your crow's feet are.

- Amazing Cosmetics Amazing Concealer
- Christopher Drummond Duo Phase Concealer
- Boots No. 7 Quick Cover Blemish Stick
- Vapour Illusionist Concealer

Powder

Tip: Be careful not to apply loose powder formulations when your baby is in the room. A lot of times more powder ends up in the air than on your brush, and it could irritate a baby's lungs.

- Koh Gen Do Natural Lighting Powder

Lips

Tip: We like our lip color to look a little imperfect. Smudge it on with your fingers and press your lips together. The worst place for lipstick to end up is at the corners of your mouth.

- Intelligent Nutrients Lip Delivery Antioxidant Gloss in Purple Maze
- Zuzu Luxe: Innocence (perfect neutral lip shade)
- Zuzu Luxe: Fraise-Light (fucshia pink with cool blue undertones)

Eyes

This tip comes from Laura Geller: "Whether you just line the top or do the whole eye, eyeliner brings back the shape—especially if your eyes are puffy or tired. The last thing you want is for them to wash into the rest of your face. What separates them and makes them look like they're lifted out and up is eyeliner."

- Urban Decay 24/7 Eye Shadow Pencil in Sin
- Kjar Weis Eyeshadow
- INIKA Eyeliner
- INIKA Mineral Eye Shadow

- Gabriel Cosmetics Long-Lasting Kohl Eye Liner
- Lavera Volumizing Mascara

Blush and Bronzer

Tip: When you're pressed for time—which is basically every day when you become a mom—sweep a little bronzer or blush on your eyelids. It works wonders!

- Josie Maran Argan Cream Blush
- Josie Maran Argan Bronzing Powder
- Tarte Mineral Powder Bronzer
- W3LL People Mineral Bronzer

Motherhood: A New Chapter in Makeup

Welcome to motherhood, where time is the ultimate luxury. Pre-baby, you might have enjoyed putting on a full face of makeup or luxuriating in the bath without any interruptions, but now that baby has arrived, you're in for a rude awakening. Not caring what you look like after you have kids is an easy trap to fall into, and one that we admittedly have dipped a toe into more than a few times. But according to new research,[4] wearing makeup gives you a leg up on likability, attractiveness, competence, and even trustworthiness. In two studies, viewers were asked to rate the same female face with and without color cosmetics. The faces were shown to a group of people for 250 milliseconds and another group of people for an unlimited amount of time. In both groups, the faces with at least a little makeup had "significant positive effects on all outcomes." The meaning? Makeup really can make a difference in your relationships.

When you're a new mom, it matters less about who you're trying to impress. But we can speak from experience when we say that

My Mommy Makeup Strategy: A Note from Melissa

I have a nine-month-old and a three-year-old, and there are days (many of them, in fact) when I feel as though I don't have enough time to apply even a swipe of mascara. The extra seconds it would take not only to place the mascara wand on my lashes and put the tube away but then make the time commitment to removing it at the end of the day sometimes seem like too much to handle.

As a new mom, it's easy to feel guilty about stealing some "me" time for yourself. But makeup time doesn't have to be "me" time if you don't want it to be. Use this time to interact with your baby. Invest in a bouncy seat to put the baby in while you put on your makeup. Make funny faces at him while you smooth on your foundation or blast the music and bop along to Madonna as you dab on the concealer. (This is a surefire way to amuse a baby—especially if your dance moves are anything like mine.)

even a splash of bronzer on your face during those grueling newborn months really makes you feel a lot better about your state. And as the study proved, makeup also makes you appear more likable. When you're a new mom struggling to push a stroller through a heavy door, trust us when we say, you'll be relying on the kindness of strangers for help. That's where you can really benefit from looking even a teeny bit more likable!

In reality, yes, it's true that, as a mom, you will always be pressed for time, but the assumption that you don't have enough time to apply makeup is just a mind-set. "There's no such thing as having no time. There's always someone busier than me, and they make time," says makeup artist Laura Geller, who, with a top-selling makeup line, a thriving store in New York City, and regular appearances on QVC, is one of the busiest moms we know.

Forget about doing a full face of makeup—those days are over! Applying your makeup as a mom shouldn't take more than five minutes because, frankly, getting all dolled up to take the kids to the park just looks weird. "There's a definite makeup look when you're running around with your kids," says Geller. "That look is clean and polished. You're mostly getting rid of dark circles and making sure that your features look a little bit more defined."

The makeup products you want to be using as a new mama are multitasking, foolproof, moisturizing, and luminizing. "I think a lot of new moms make the mistake of doing too heavy of a makeup look to compensate for looking tired," says author and beauty expert Lois Joy Johnson. "I love highlighter pens and pencils for adding a fresh look. Use them at the inner and outer corners of the eye. You want to keep the sparkle there, so go for shimmery eye shadows—not metallic or glitter—but shimmery to make your eyes look awake and alive."

Another key to feeling good is not feeling guilty about spending time or money on yourself instead of your baby. "I'm floored by the amount of paraphernalia moms have for their children and almost nothing for themselves," says Johnson, who raised two daughters while working full-time as a beauty editor at glossy magazines. We couldn't agree more. Our homes are filled to the rafters with a rainbow array of puzzles, stuffed animals, and strollers for every occasion. Rather than blowing $100 on another toy or outfit for your six-month-old—something he or she will surely grow out of in a matter of weeks—spend a little money on a new foundation, a pretty neutral shade of eye shadow, a manicure, or a new haircut. "I think it's important to stay connected to that part of yourself that feels sexy and sensual and likes looking attractive. Don't fall into the trap of thinking just because you had a baby it's okay to look like a hag." We can't stress this enough: happy mom = happy baby!

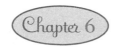

Staying Smart at the Salon and Spa

Nails, Hair, Massage, and More

Just as we don't expect you to go cold turkey with your beauty products, we would never tell any mom-to-be to cancel all her spa and salon appointments for nine months. We certainly didn't do that. We both continued coloring our hair and indulging in manis and pedis as well as facials and massages. Gray hair, five-inch dark roots, and ratty fingernails don't need to become the telltale signs that you've got a bun in the oven. In fact, looking like a million bucks when you may only be feeling like a five-spot can do a lot for the psyche. In our opinion, there's nothing like looking down at perfectly painted nails in a brilliant shade of coral or a chic taupe hue to boost the spirit and make you feel put together—even if the rest of you feels bloated or exhausted.

As we've been saying, it's important to exercise caution during pregnancy, and the spa and salon are no exception. Hair color has long been a topic of debate in terms of safety during pregnancy, and we'll talk more about that later, but there are some other precautions to take when heading out for your beauty services that you may not be aware of. We will fill you in on everything you need to know before you get to the salon so you can relax while you're there and not have to worry about walking out with a nasty infection from a dirty footbath. Thankfully, there are smarter ways to color your hair and get pedicures during pregnancy. As in all of the other chapters, we're presenting you with a third option that falls somewhere between boycotting the salon and spa during pregnancy and just sticking with your pre-pregnancy regimen—a beauty compromise.

Mom-Smarts on Hair Color

To Color or Not to Color?

Coloring your hair is a lightning rod topic among pregnant women. We know many women who say, "Forget it," and let their grays come out of hiding or their dark roots grow to their chins. Others choose to exercise caution and wait until the second trimester to pay a visit to the salon, and yet others refuse to let their locks look anything less than spectacular and stick to their normal coloring routine. "There's no data to support that coloring your hair is harmful to mom or baby," says Dr. Abel, a perinatologist at the Deaconess Medical Center in Spokane, Washington. In fact, Dr. Abel says, he's more concerned about the fumes a pregnant woman might encounter at the salon than about the color sitting on her hair. "I tell my patients to make sure they're in a salon that's well ventilated. I don't want them passing out and hitting their head from the fumes," he says.

Something to keep in mind is that hair itself is a dead fiber. "Hair is made of keratin and has no life force of its own," says celebrity hairstylist and salon owner Eva Scrivo. "Whatever comes

in contact with your hair does not get absorbed into your body."
Your hair may not be alive, but your scalp definitely is. And while
it's true that research hasn't shown that coloring your hair is
harmful during pregnancy, Dr. Rubin cautions, "There are hundreds of ingredients used in different hair color products, and
some of them do have links to harmful effects on the fetus in sep-
arate studies."

So what to do? We were confused too. The Organization of
Teratology Information Specialists states that "low levels of hair
dye can be absorbed through the skin after application, and the
dye is excreted into the urine. This minimal amount is not thought
to be enough to cause a problem for the baby." No studies of the
effects of hair dyes on the fetus have been done, since it's considered unethical to conduct certain kinds of experiments on pregnant humans, but common sense tells us that laying off the heavy
color treatments that sit on the scalp is the way to go. OTIS also
states: "One study found a slightly increased risk for miscarriage
for cosmetologists who had specific work activities. Activities that
seemed to contribute to the slightly increased risk included working more than 40 hours per week, standing more than eight hours
per day, higher numbers of bleaches and permanents applied per
week, and working in salons where nail sculpturing was per-
formed." So, in other words, it's hard to say exactly whether it was
the stress of working hard or the chemicals themselves that
caused these miscarriages.

Referring to another study, OTIS also notes that "miscarriage
rates among hairdressers were reviewed, and newer data was com-
pared to older data. The older data [from 1986 to 1988] showed an
increased risk of miscarriage, an extended time trying to get pregnant, and low birth weight. The newer data [from 1991 to 1993]
did not find increased risks." That's good news for those who work

in the cosmetology business. Even so, there are still powerful chemicals inside hair dyes, and we decided to err on the side of caution. Since it's hard to see what's really going on under the hair on your head—for example, what if you had a cut or a scrape on your scalp that you couldn't see?—we didn't want to create an open door for chemicals to seep in. (Later in the chapter, see our "Do Not Use" list of the chemicals to steer clear of at the salon.)

We believe that highlights and lowlights—basically any color that does not sit on the scalp—are a good choice during pregnancy. Vegetable-based colors are another good option, but they're not for everyone, especially those people (ahem, like us) who want to be sure they walk away with a hair color they like. "The problem with vegetable-based colors is that they are hard to control, meaning that the color you chose isn't always the color that you get," explains Scrivo. "They may oxidize and turn into a different shade than the one you chose. Typically vegetable-based colors are warmer because they're not professionally made and the color is not stabilized."

The Truth About "Backbar" Products

Finding out every single ingredient that goes into your hair color at the salon may be a mission impossible, because companies that make products not intended for retail sale (aka "backbar" products) are not required to list their ingredients.

Cosmetics produced or distributed for retail sale to consumers for their personal care are required to bear an ingredient declaration. Cosmetics not customarily distributed for retail sale, e.g., hair preparations or make-up products used by professionals on customers at their establishments and skin cleansing or emollient creams used by persons at their places of work, are exempt from this requirement provided these products are not also sold to consumers at professional establishments or workplaces for their consumption at home.[1]

Our suggestion? Ask your colorist what the ingredients are in your hair color preparation so as to alert you to the presence of any chemicals you're hoping to avoid. If your colorist doesn't know the ingredients and you can't find any information about them any other way, then considering that the product is going to sit on your scalp or be inhaled into your lungs, it's probably safer to wait until after pregnancy to use it.

Say "Heck No" to Henna

"One of the biggest misconceptions is that henna is good for the hair," says Scrivo. Henna comes from the dried leaves of a plant. It's natural, but it forms a hard coating on the hair and is very difficult, if not impossible, to remove. The hard coating doesn't allow other good things like masks, conditioners, natural oils, or hair color to penetrate. If you want to go back to coloring your hair normally after your pregnancy, it won't be able to penetrate the henna. So you'll either have to get a major haircut to get rid of the henna or end up with two-toned hair. Scrivo says that henna is not worth the long-term havoc it wreaks on hair.

Skip Coloring in the First Trimester

The first trimester is a time when critical neurological development is going on inside your baby. Think about the fact that he or she is going from a few tiny cells to a breathing human being. It's not a time when you want to take any chances. There are smart options for covering silver strands while carrying a baby. "It comes down to ammonia-free or vegetable-based color," says Scrivo. "My personal

My Pregnancy Hair Color Strategy: A Note from Melissa

I highlighted my hair through both pregnancies but waited until the second trimester, just to be on the safe side. My preferred method is balayage (aka hair painting). It's highlighting sans the foils, so there's no telltale sign screaming: "Hey, I color my hair!" I also did an ammonia-free gloss in between balayage sessions during my last pregnancy. It gave my color a gorgeous boost and left my hair ridiculously glossy. Plus, it was quick and didn't smell at all. The gloss allowed me to let my highlights grow out longer than usual through the duration of my pregnancy. Rather than getting a touch-up every eight weeks, I waited almost four months between highlights. Because the way that balayaged hair grows out, I was left with cool ombre surfer-girl hair—a look I loved so much that I now continue to get highlights every four months. It's much healthier for my hair and saves a lot of money too. Another thing I loved about getting my hair done during pregnancy? Those amazing scalp massages while getting my hair shampooed. They did wonders for my awful hormone-induced headaches.

recommendation is not doing it in the first trimester, but waiting until the second trimester and using ammonia-free color."

Ask for Ammonia-Free Color

Why exactly do we want to avoid ammonia in our hair color? Besides the nasty fumes it gives off, ammonia is also the culprit behind scalp itchiness and inflammation, coughing, and difficulty breathing. These are all symptoms you want to avoid, pregnant or not. Ammonia also opens the cuticle of the hair quickly and widely

---

Try This at Home

Couture Colour is a new ammonia-free at-home coloring system that uses oil from the pequi fruit (found in the Amazon rain forest) to gently open the cuticle and MEA to push the pigments into the hair. Coloring your hair at home is a great option for moms-to-be—just think of all the potential fumes from a busy salon you'll be avoiding. If you want to be extra cautious about inhalation, color your hair outside.

---

to allow the color to penetrate. Once that happens, the cuticle doesn't lie as flat anymore, creating frizziness and hair that's not as soft as it was pre-color.

Recently companies have stepped up to the plate and started coming out with formulas that do not contain ammonia. One at the forefront of this movement is INOA from L'Oreal Professionel. INOA, which stands for Innovation No Ammonia, uses MEA (mono-ethanolamine), which is gentler and kinder than ammonia, as its alkalizing agent, at the same percentage found in a glaze. Unlike ammonia, MEA opens the cuticle only halfway. INOA came out with a special oil-delivery system that helps the MEA push the color into the hair. Not only is your hair receiving benefits from the oil, but it's also getting a much gentler treatment that involves minimal cuticle abuse. A win-win situation if you ask us! Check out the L'Oreal Professionel website (www.inoa-us.com) to find a salon near you that offers INOA.

Try a Glaze

If you color your hair, you're probably aware of glazes. They are *demi-permanent,* meaning that they use a different alkalizing agent

Salon Treatments

Do Use

- Ammonia-free color
- Highlights or foils
- Balayage (hair painting)
- Vegetable-based colors

Do Not Use

- *Any hair color containing the chemical paraphenylenediamine (PPD),* which is most often an ingredient in permanent black hair dyes. PPD has been found to cause severe allergic reactions and, in rare cases, death.
- *Formaldehyde,* a colorless gas with an extremely strong odor. It's been in the news recently because it was found in the popular Brazilian hair-straightening treatments. It's considered a "probable human carcinogen," and exposure is thought to be linked to sperm damage and spontaneous abortion.[2]
- *Any straightening or permanent treatment containing keratin,* which may contain formaldehyde or formaldehyde derivatives.

than ammonia. Glazes give the hair a boost of shine and a wash of color. They are a great way to cover grays or to give your natural hair color a little oomph. Again, the alkalizing agent used is MEA. "The reason it's called a 'glaze' is because it's left on for a fraction of the time as permanent color," says Scrivo. After only one to ten minutes, the glaze is washed off. When you're pregnant, knowing that the color is staying on your hair for such a short amount of time is a relief.

Speak Up at the Salon!

Melissa's family is always telling her: "Be your own advocate." That means, speak up when something doesn't feel right. One place you definitely want to speak out is at the salon. If the smell is bringing tears to your eyes, or you want to move chairs to be closer to an open window or door, don't be afraid to speak up! Hairdressers are not mind-readers. If you're afraid of being impolite, don't forget that the most important thing is the growing baby inside you, not your hair colorist's feelings. If you're worried about inhaling fumes, then wait until the second trimester, and no matter when you go, make sure the salon is well ventilated.

Scrivo advises asking whether the salon does keratin straightening treatments, "and if so, is there a day they don't do those treatments or can you sit away from those treatments in progress? Keratin treatments sometimes contain formaldehyde, which is a vapor that lifts off the hair and becomes a gas in the room." And research studies show links to birth defects in the children of women who were exposed to formaldehyde in the workplace during the first trimester (along with other chemicals).

Ask your colorist to give you a seat near the door or to let you crack open a window. If you feel like you're breathing in chemicals, then guess what? You probably are. If you're sitting next to someone doing a chemical relaxer or a perm, then ask politely to be moved. If the salon can't accommodate you, then you can always come back later—or find another salon!

Mom-Smart Nails

We've always found manicures and pedicures to be instant mood-lifters. Who doesn't feel just a little bit more put together and

---

**Stress and Pregnancy:
Or, Why We're Forgoing the Brazilian Bikini Waxes!**

Research shows that high levels of stress and anxiety during pregnancy are associated with the development of ADHD with poor impulse control later in the child's life (age eight to nine years). Severe stress has also been linked to miscarriage, premature delivery, and low birth weight. We're not saying that a Brazilian bikini wax will definitely give your son ADHD, but what we are saying is that avoiding any kind of stress, whether physical or emotional—including having the hair ripped from your nether regions—is a good idea during pregnancy.

---

glamorous when her nails are clean, shaped, and painted to perfection? That's why we'd never tell you to forgo a visit to the nail salon or to leave your nails unattended to for nine months. But we do want to arm you with the knowledge to make your manis and pedis as safe as possible.

It's easy to think of nails as strong barriers that shield any and all bacteria, but that's actually not the case. "Your fingernail under a microscope looks like a piece of wood," says Nonie Crème, founder of the hip nail care line Butter London. "It's layers and layers of long strands of fiber. They are absolutely porous. Why do you think your nails get bendy if you stay in the bathtub for too long?" Which is why we need to worry about what goes onto our fingernails as much as we think about what goes onto other areas of our body.

Check the Label on Your Nail Polish

Let's start with the actual nail polish. Until recently, most nail polishes contained three nasty ingredients: DBP (dibutyl phthalate), toluene, and formaldehyde. While fortunately safer formulations have been created, unfortunately many nail polishes on the market and at the salon still contain these nasties. Toluene is linked to birth defects and human reproductive and developmental problems; formaldehyde, as discussed earlier, is a carcinogen and an indoor air pollutant with links to birth defects; and phthalates have been linked to birth defects as well. So, needless to say, these are three chemicals we'd rather not be painting onto our nails during pregnancy—or any other time for that matter.

Nonie Crème felt the same way, which is one of the reasons she created Butter London, a line that helped coin the term "3-Free" (as in, free of those three nasties). Crème, a native Brit, makes sure that all her products pass the more rigid European Union (EU) safety standards. "The US is literally referred to as the 'Wild West' in terms of beauty," she says. "Lacquer is still a highly chemical product, and we'll probably never be able to make them out of watercolor, but what I can promise you is that we are about ethics, and it's unethical to put poison in your products."

Even more important than choosing nail color that's 3-Free is going with a 3-Free base coat, since that layer goes directly onto the nail plate. Plus, as Crème points out, 3-Free and non-3-Free polishes dry at different rates: if you use a non-3-Free base or top coat, you can expect your polish to peel off the next day.

Our Favorite 3-Free Nail Polish Lines

- *Butter London:* Nails become major style statements thanks to Crème's London fashion industry roots. Yummy Mummy— a taupey-beige shade—looks good on everyone. "It's our best-selling product—we call it the 'magic lacquer' because it hides a multitude of sins!" says Crème.

- *RGB:* We love the rich, neutral colors from this ultra-modern, well-edited collection of nail polishes. Their chic, fashion-forward shades get tons of editorial play and celebrity shout-outs.
- *Zoya:* From creamy nude shades to mod mattes and fun metallics, there's something for everyone in Zoya's range of over three hundred colors. Founded in 1986, Zoya was the first line to remove toxic ingredients such as toluene, camphor, formaldehyde, and DBP from its formulations.
- *Lippmann Collection:* Deborah Lippmann is the celebrity manicurist behind this line of ultra-cool colors. Her genius colors often come from collaborations with fashion designers and celebrities. Lippmann Collection is always a presence backstage at runway shows and on fashion shoots. We love Glamorous Life, a metallic rose-gold shade inspired by Rolex watches.
- *Essie:* Our favorite nail salon brand has gone 3-Free too. We love Essie polishes for their witty names and awesome colors. Sugar Daddy is our go-to manicure shade.
- *NARS:* For high-fashion colors, we rely on the NARS collection of brilliant shades and formulations. They have some of the best pedicure colors around! We made sure to get our toes painted right before our due dates. Somehow a bright and perfect pedicure made the whole hospital experience a little more glamorous.
- *Revlon:* We were thrilled to learn that Revlon, one of our favorite drugstore brands, went 3-Free. The colors in this line are literally limitless!

Nail Salon Safety

We've all heard the stories about some poor woman getting a wart, a blister, or a staph infection at the nail salon. There's no worse time to contract one of these ailments than during pregnancy, when your defenses are down and your treatment options are limited. To make your manicures and pedicures safer, forgo the finger bowl and the foot spa. "You don't need them. What you need is for someone to sterilize your skin with a hand sanitizer or wash the hands thoroughly," says Crème. It's impossible to know if those bowls have been washed properly or if any of the clients who used them before you were sick.

Butter London's nail spa in Seattle is completely waterless. Crème explains why: "The way the foot spa filtration system works is like a bathtub drain. They file your foot and all of the dead skin cells, all the yucky, goes in the water, and they simply pull the drain and all of the muck drains away. Just like in a bathtub, those foot spa drains get very clogged with dead skin way deep into the filtration system where you can't even see it. It doesn't matter how much they bleach the foot spa—every time they fill the basin that filth that is blocking the drain pops back up through the drain, so you're soaking your feet in hundreds of people's rotten muck. If you have a dodgy toenail or an open cut, imagine all that bacteria from the foot spa going into that wound."

If that's not enough graphic info to persuade you to forgo the foot spa, then consider the fact that the American Academy of Dermatology lists among pedicure health risks fungal infections and bacterial skin infections, including the antibiotic-resistant infection MRSA (methicillin-resistant staphylococcus aureus).

Leave Your Cuticles Alone!

We've all been there. You go in for a manicure, and you've got some messy hangnails and ragged-looking cuticles. When the manicurist starts snipping the cuticles, you can't bring yourself to tell her to stop. After all, what's the harm of a little trim job? A lot, as it turns

Be Smart at the Nail Salon

The last thing you want during pregnancy is a nasty bacterial infection! Don't be afraid to be high-maintenance at the salon. Go through this checklist before you head out for your next mani/pedi.

- Bring your own 3-Free color, including top and base coats.
- Tell the manicurist not to cut your cuticles—just push them back.
- Ask to go waterless—no foot spas and no finger bowls.
- If you must use a foot spa, ask whether it's been disinfected.
- Don't shave right before a pedicure.
- Don't get a pedicure if you have any open wounds on your feet or legs.
- Go to the salon early. Pedicure instruments are cleanest at the beginning of the day.
- Forgo the aerosol can of quick dry, which is loaded with chemicals that can easily enter the lungs; instead, let your nails air-dry.

out. "Your cuticle exists as a seal—it forms a seal over the nail bed to stop infection and germs from getting in," explains Crème. "When you chop that off, you'll notice that your fingers hurt and ache afterwards. The reason they ache is because you have all this microscopic bacteria and germs sitting in your nail bed. Then when the cuticle grows back, you've got a big fat ridge where the nail was fighting infection."

As it turns out, cutting the cuticle is a vicious cycle. When you cut the cuticle off, your body thinks it's been injured, so your brain sends a message to your body to rev up skin cell production, leading to cuticles that grow back even thicker than they were. The situation, however, is not hopeless. "Through gentle and consistent exfoliation, where you're just exfoliating the dead skin off the top, you can retrain your cuticles to grow back thin and soft and small," says Crème.

Mom-Smart Facials

Getting a facial is the skin equivalent of going to the dentist for a professional teeth cleaning. A good facial will deep-clean your pores and leave your skin looking and feeling refreshed and glowing. We're both big advocates of facials. Some facials come with lots of bells and whistles, such as electric currents, chemical peels, or light therapies, but when you're pregnant it's best to stick with a basic facial that does no more than give your skin a good cleaning without the use of lasers or chemicals.

"More times than not, skin care concerns are magnified during pregnancy and must be treated naturally and without chemicals," says celebrity facialist Kate Somerville, whose clients include celebrity moms Jessica Alba and Debra Messing. At Kate Somerville Skin Health Experts Clinic, her famous Los Angeles skin clinic, she offers a pregnancy facial, created specifically to deal with mom-related skin issues like hormone fluctuations, dehydration, and puffiness and steers clear of any ingredients that could be harmful to the baby. "For example, if a woman is suffering from pigmentation, we'll treat the skin with vitamin C, which brightens and lightens, since we can't turn to chemicals like hydroquinone or retinols. We also avoid lasers, vitamin A, or retinols," she says. Dr. Macrene Alexiades-Armenakas agrees: "Absolutely avoid laser or electric currents of any kind during pregnancy, as they are contraindicated and could potentially cause hyperpigmentation, which is more common during pregnancy due to hormones."

One of the things we love—and hate—about facials is extractions. While they hurt like hell, they get rid of any nascent pimples we have waiting to pop out. But are they safe during pregnancy? "Extractions are safe in expert hands, and only if not done too deeply," advises Dr. Alexiades-Armenakas. She recommends letting an experienced dermatologist do the job.

If you want a completely pregnancy-safe way to give yourself a mini-facial, try steaming your face at home. Steaming loosens dirt, unclogs pores, and deeply cleans your face. It's super easy too— here's how to do it:

- Boil some water and remove it from the stove.
- Drape a towel over your head to keep steam from escaping.
- Stand with your face over the bowl for about ten minutes.

Another thing to keep in mind is that, thanks to all of those extra hormones that have made themselves at home inside your body, your skin will be much more sensitive during pregnancy. A standard facial might turn out to be a wholly unpleasant experience, especially if extractions are involved. Make sure to tell your facialist if the pressure is just too much to bear and ask for a light head massage if it becomes too painful.

Mom-Smart Massage

There might be no better time in your life to indulge in a massage than when you're pregnant. We know how sore and uncomfortable pregnancy can be and how muscles you didn't even know you had can ache. "Structurally everything in your body is different. Your shape has changed, your rib cage has expanded, and your pelvis has widened," says prenatal massage therapist Janet Markovits. "Mas-

Ask Dr. Rubin

Q: *I have chemical peels done at my spa every month to control my acne. Should I continue them while I am pregnant?*

A: It depends on which kind you are using. Chemical peels come in several varieties and contain one or more *keratolytics,* or chemicals that soften the epidermis, unclog pores, and remove layers of dead skin cells. Many of the commonly available peels use ingredients such as salicylic acid and glycolic acid that have links to birth defects in published medical studies. Lactic acid, however, is a highly effective keratolytic that passes through teratology screening cleanly because it is already naturally found in your body. It also happens to be less irritating to the skin than other peels.

sage helps with everything from constipation and headaches to anxiety and, of course, muscle pain."

The benefits of massage are not up for debate, but nevertheless, you might have heard that massages are not safe during the first trimester. Not true, says Markovits. "Many spas have a rule against therapists working on someone during the first trimester, but their reasoning has to do with lawsuits and litigation," she says. "They're afraid that if someone miscarries, then they'll be liable, but massage does not cause miscarriage—it's a huge misconception."

One thing you don't want to do during a massage is lie flat on your back. After eighteen weeks of pregnancy, the uterus becomes very heavy, and if you're lying flat on your back you increase the chances of it compressing the vena cava blood vessel, which could cause a drop in blood pressure. Make sure that the massage table either has a cutout for your belly, so you can lie on your stomach, or that you are propped up on your left side with pillows surrounding you. Personally, we find the side position to be the most comfortable.

You also need to make sure the massage therapist is certified. "When you're pregnant, you really want to go to somebody certified in pregnancy massage," says Markovits. "If you go to somebody who is not trained, then they're not familiar with all of the different things that are going on in your body." When you're pregnant, your blood volume is elevated, which could lead to blood clots, something the masseuse needs to be aware of. Another pregnancy-specific issue is swollen legs. "When there's swelling in the legs, you actually want the massage to be pretty light and not very deep with the pressure because that water level layer is on the very top superficial layer and if you go any deeper it completely bypasses it," says Markovits. "If you go to someone not trained, they might give you a really deep massage to the legs, which is not the best thing when you're pregnant." To find a trained massage therapist in your area, go to the Mother Massage website (www.mothermassage.net).

Nine months is a long time to go without indulging in a beauty treatment—even for women like us, who are on the low-maintenance side. We wouldn't feel quite like ourselves if we left our nails unkempt and unpainted. Our time at the salon and spa is also a sacred ritual, something that neither of us has given up even after having children. In fact, each of us made a first venture out into the real world after having a baby by going to the hair salon to get those grays touched up.

"Nobody talks about the recovery time once you've had the baby. Take your family and friends up on the help they offer and get some rest when you can," advises Kate Somerville. "Do something for yourself—women tend to nourish the baby, take care of their husband and the house. When you do take the time for yourself, do a mask or get your nails done. The tiny bit you do benefits everyone."

We couldn't agree more. We do some of our best thinking when we make time for ourselves. We leave the spa feeling more re-freshed and ready to take on the day. Motherhood is the hardest—and most rewarding—job there is. We fully believe that treating yourself to some spa time is part of the deal.

Baby-Smart Skin Care

I t would seem logical that products marketed for babies are in fact safe for babies, right? Sadly, that's not the case. "I was shocked by what I found in baby skin care products, especially from a lot of the popular brands," says Tami Main, founder of Taslie Skincare, a baby-smart line she created when she became a mom. She's referring to some of the best-known names in the baby care business. Many of them are the same brands our moms used on us when we were babies. Some of these brands use ingredients that have been recognized as carcinogens, such as 1,4-dioxane and quaternium-15, and many of them contain hormone-mimicking chemicals and artificial fragrances, which, as you'll learn in this chapter, are other red flags for babies.

The baby products business is a nearly $8.1 billion industry. That's a lot of wipes, toys, and gadgets. While there are many totally safe, genius inventions on the market, there are also a lot of products that we just don't have enough information on to deem completely safe.

The United States imports or produces about 27 trillion pounds of chemicals each year. The primary law that regulates these chemicals is the Toxic Substances Control Act (TSCA). When the law was first passed in 1976, 62,000 chemicals were allowed to remain on the market without any testing of their effects on health or the environment. In the years since the law was passed, only about 200 chemicals have been tested. Under the current law, instead of testing chemicals for safety before they hit the market, the Environmental Protection Agency (EPA) must prove that there's an "unreasonable risk" before they can be regulated. The American Academy of Pediatrics (AAP) recently issued a statement that the TSCA "fails to protect children and pregnant women." The AAP made a list of recommendations for the TSCA, which has not been updated in over thirty-five years, including: "Make chemical testing relevant to the special needs of pregnant women and children, by including data on reproductive and developmental toxicity, including endocrine disruption, as it relates to reproduction, neurotoxicity, and puberty."[1]

With the lack of action by Congress, more action has to be taken by parents. As parents, we must be aware that we cannot rely on antiquated lists of chemicals that have not been properly policed by our government. It's important that we take the initiative and read the ingredient labels on our children's products to determine ourselves whether or not they are safe. It's a job no one else is going to do for us.

Because our children's skin is more delicate and sensitive than ours, they are more susceptible to absorbing harmful ingredients. "Baby skin is virgin skin," says pediatric dermatologist Robin Schaffran. "Things get absorbed much more easily into a newborn's skin." When it comes to topical ingredient safety, the rules of the game change a bit for babies versus pregnant women. Nobody of any age wants to use chemicals with links to cancer, but with an infant it's also really important to avoid ingredients that have estrogenic effects. Those agents are called xenoestrogens.

Xenoestrogens are a group of natural and man-made chemicals that behave very similarly to estrogen. Why don't we want xenoestrogens in our baby's skin care products? The plain and simple explanation is that they disrupt the hormonal balance in both genders. Remember that study on tea tree and lavender oils we told you about earlier? And how these ingredients are thought to cause breast growth in male children? Well, xenoestrogens are also thought to cause the early onset of puberty in girls, so it's extremely important to avoid them from infancy through puberty.

The topical xenoestrogens we know of include the paraben class of preservatives, the chemical class of sunscreens, phthalates, dichlorodiphenyltrichloroethane (DDT) pesticide, lavender, tea tree oil, and soy. Parabens, which are preservatives used in many baby lotions and washes, are potential endocrine disrupters. They are banned in Denmark for use in products for kids under the age of three. Phthalates are found in products with synthetic fragrances. They've been connected with low sperm quality, among other genital disorders, in males, as well as with early onset of puberty in girls. Their use has been restricted in children's toys since 2008, but they're still found in many personal care products. You won't find phthalates on most ingredient lists, so refer to our "Reduce Your Use" list later in this chapter to find out how to decipher them. Lavender, tea tree oil, and soy are considered "natural" ingredients, but even so, case reports have linked them to possible estrogenic effects. While these ingredients have no proven risks for pregnant women or other adults, their hormone-like effects may disrupt normal hormonal activity in boys who have not yet reached puberty. A few case reports suggest that they cause abnormal breast growth in boys, a condition known as gynecomastia. Chemical sunscreen ingredients, including oxybenzone and avobenzone (see "Reduce Your Use" for all the other ingredients), are commonly found in sun care products deemed "safe" for baby. Well, they're not. They all have shown estrogenic effects, and since they are absorbed into the skin, these are not ingredients you want to use on babies.

Other ingredients you want to be aware of are the carcinogens in baby products. The most common ones used in baby personal care products are 1,4-dioxane, a by-product of a process that makes chemicals gentler to the skin, and quaternium-15, a bacteria-killing preservative that releases formaldehyde.

Why Some Ingredients Should Irritate You— and Your Baby

Up to 30 percent of children will suffer from eczema, dermatitis, or sensitive skin at some point. So besides the xenoestrogens, we also need to be aware of irritating ingredients. "The most obvious irritants are fragrances, colors, and, for many, nut oils, including natural ingredients such as shea butter," says John Gardiner, CEO of Exederm, a gentle line of skin care products made for kids with skin allergies and eczema.

Remember how we said in Chapter 1 that the terms "organic" and "natural" can be misleading? Well, the same is true with the words "hypoallergenic" and "sensitive." "Unfortunately, the phrases 'hypoallergenic' and 'sensitive' are often abused, and there are no rules or regulations governing their use—anyone can claim to be hypoallergenic," says Gardiner. "This is why it's important to try to read the label or check with a medical professional." Whether it's diaper rash or eczema, dealing with baby skin issues isn't fun for either the baby or the parent. Gardiner advises checking the website of groups like the National Eczema Association (www.easeeczema.org) for answers to questions you may have about the baby products you want to use.

Another word you want to steer clear of on labels is "fragrance." "Fragrances in general are a no-no in my world for babies," says Dr.

Schaffran. Ironically, it's that "new baby smell" that lures many moms to buy baby products loaded with fragrance. Who doesn't love that sweet baby scent? It's basically instilled in us early in life, even if it's not representative of what a baby actually smells like. One of our favorite perfumes as teenagers was Love's Baby Soft, which mimicked the innocent, powdery aroma associated with babies. It was so popular back then that our junior high school hallways reeked of the stuff. That cloying scent can also be found in a myriad of lotions, deodorants, and other perfumes.

But here's the funny part—real babies don't smell like that. Their natural scent isn't sweet and powdery at all. They have more of a real human smell, minus the postpubescent body odor. Don't get us wrong, we loved the way our babies smelled, mainly because they were our babies and whatever odor they produced would have smelled like fresh-baked cookies to us. Even dried-up drool, poop, spit-up, and milk trapped in their neck folds for days didn't smell as bad to us as it might have to a stranger. One of the reasons is that it's thought that babies produce a special scent that helps strengthen the parent-baby bond. A study conducted at Lund University in Sweden in 2001 found that a distinct baby smell acts like a pheromone to help new parents bond with their babies. Our thought is, why mess with that natural odor? The last thing we want to do is thwart the amazing power of Mother Nature by masking natural smells with synthetic fragrances, especially if they're detrimental.

"Fragrance in products is just not necessary and can be extremely irritating," says Dr. Schaffran. Her recommendation is to use a drop of essential oil on your baby if you really want him or her to have a scent. Dr. Rubin feels that small amounts of synthetic fragrance can be okay, "as long as you know that the product is free of phthalates and has passed irritation and allergy testing.

Remember—many natural, fragrant essential oils cause irritation and allergies too," he says. To make sure the product is phthalate-free, look for the label to say as much.

Regardless of what you decide to put on your baby, the last thing you want is for your little one to have an allergic reaction, so be sure to perform a patch test first. "Apply a small dab of product to the underside of their arm, once daily, for three days in a row," says Dr. Rubin. "If there is no redness or irritation on the fourth day, then it's probably okay to use the product as directed."

Clothes Call

Another area you may need to make over before baby arrives is the laundry room. Just as fragranced topical products might irritate your munchkin's sensitive skin, blankets and clothing washed in scented laundry detergents can do the same thing. It's best to take the safe route and switch to a detergent free of fragrance and dyes. Be forewarned that when you use a fragrance-free detergent, your baby's laundry won't have the "fresh and clean" smell to it anymore, but we feel it's the smarter bet. We'll take unscented onesies over giving our baby a rash any day of the week.

Also be sure to wash any clothing, blankets, or cloth diapers before you put them on your baby. You don't know where these items have been before you bought them, and an item purchased at a store is especially likely to have had lots of fingers touching it before yours. Also, many manufacturers apply a fabric finisher to clothing, which could irritate your baby's skin. Our advice? Order all of your baby clothes and accessories online to cut down on the number of people who may have tried them on or handled them.

Here's our list of the baby-smart laundry detergents we use and love:

- BabyGanics Loads of Love Fragrance-Free Laundry Detergent (www.babyganics.com): We are huge BabyGanics fans, and their fragrance-free laundry detergent just makes us even more excited about the brand. Because it's three times more concentrated than a typical detergent, it really gets the stains out—but using nontoxic ingredients. We love that you can pretreat stains with it, which comes in handy when your baby poops and spits up all over himself multiple times a day.
- Tide Free and Gentle (www.tide.com): Melissa grew up on Tide, so this has been her go-to detergent ever since her first son was born. After using it on both kids for over three years, she can report that neither of them has ever developed a rash or irritation from their clothes.
- Seventh Generation Baby Laundry Detergent (www.seventhgeneration .com): Seventh Generation is another great brand we have deep respect for. Its Baby Laundry Detergent uses enzymes rather than harsh agents to lift stains. The formula is biodegradable, so it will also appeal to your environmentally conscious side.

The Most Common Baby Skin Care Concerns

Every mom-to-be daydreams about what it's going to be like cuddling up to her newborn baby. We imagined the sensation of nuzzling that flawless, downy soft skin while images of cute pinchable cheeks and perfect little tushies danced in our minds. In reality, we have both had to deal with cradle cap and eczema and will probably be waging the battle against diaper rash until our boys are finally potty-trained!

Here's the lowdown on the skin issues you too can expect to confront when your baby arrives.

Diaper Rash

What it is: You know it's diaper rash (*diaper dermatitis*) when you see a patchwork of bright redness or pimplelike dots on the area of your baby's skin underneath the diaper. Diaper rash can vary from just a little irritation to welts and dry, chapped, sometimes bleeding skin. Regardless of how mild or intense the rash looks, it can make your little one extremely uncomfortable and fussy.

The cause: Diaper rash is usually caused by the baby's sensitive skin being exposed to urine- or feces-related moisture present in the diaper for prolonged periods of time. Your baby can also get it from the friction caused by running or crawling around in the diaper. New foods are also a likely candidate. When babies are introduced to solids, their stools change, which can be irritating.

How to treat it: Change your baby's diaper often. For newborns that means every two hours. And always change poopy diapers immediately! Wet, dark places are breeding grounds for rashes and fungal infections, which can sometimes accompany diaper rash. Be sure to wipe the diaper area clean after each changing, even if it's only urine you're cleaning up. Leave the diaper off until the area is completely air-dried. Yep, that means letting your baby hang out without any diaper on for a few minutes! Just place a thick towel or pad underneath your baby to absorb any accidents. After the area is dry, apply a baby-safe diaper cream (see the end of the chapter for our recommendations) if you see any signs of irritation.

There are a few other causes of rashes in the diaper area that need to be treated with prescription medications, so if your baby's rash is severe, or it's not clearing up quickly, or you're just not sure, make an appointment with your pediatrician pronto!

Cradle Cap

What it is: Cradle cap (*seborrheic dermatitis*) is basically infant dandruff. You know your little one has it when you see white or yellow flaky scales on oily areas like the scalp, ears, or eyelids.

The cause: The cause isn't 100 percent clear, but experts think it happens when mom passes hormones to baby before birth that cause an overproduction of oil in the hair follicles.

How to treat it: Regular washing of the baby's hair and scalp should do the trick. When you give your baby a bath, first wet the head, then use a baby brush (a toothbrush works too) to brush the scalp and loosen the flakes. Next, use one of the baby-smart shampoos recommended later in this chapter and lather it up on your baby's head. Massage the scalp for a few minutes with the shampoo, then rinse. Even on the days you don't wash your baby, brush his or her hair several times a day with a soft brush or comb. One of our favorites is the wooden brush and comb set from Green Sprouts (www.iplaybabywear.com).

Eczema

What it is: This itchy rash usually rears its ugly head between the ages of two and six months. The dry, red, scaly patches typically start on the face, then spread to other areas of the body. The difference between eczema (*atopic dermatitis*) and just regular dry skin is that eczema is extremely inflamed, swollen, and sometimes crusting.

The cause: Babies can develop eczema from a multitude of sources, ranging from a family history of allergies (the "atopic" in *atopic dermatitis* indicates that it's hereditary) to environmental factors. But as with most skin allergies, you may never find out the actual cause. And that certainly can be frustrating! Babies with

Fragrance Is Not Your Breast Friend

Babies like how their mommies smell. They're not too big on masking fragrances or overpowering perfumes. Not only might those artificial scents give them a headache, an allergic reaction, or even an asthma attack, but they can also confuse babies when it comes to breast-feeding. Some babies may not latch on as easily if they taste or smell perfume. Spraying fragrance or smearing body lotion on your nipples or the surrounding area just isn't a good idea if you're breast-feeding. Alternatively, if you can't live without your fragrance, try applying only a small amount to the backs of your knees, where it's more subtle and farther away from baby's nose.

eczema also have a problem retaining moisture and are prone to dry skin.

How to treat it: There are two ways to win the war against eczema: fight suspected irritants and allergens, and keep the skin as hydrated as possible. We know some moms who made major lifestyle changes when their baby developed eczema. Even though it's hard to pinpoint the exact cause of eczema, you can take these steps to relieve your baby's symptoms:

- Cut out all fragranced products for your baby.
- Wash all new clothes before your baby wears them.
- Moisturize your baby right after bath time to lock in moisture.
- Use a water purifier for bath time (read more about this in the bath section).
- Dress your baby in only the softest clothing around and stay away from itchy, scratchy fabrics.

Reduce Your Use: Baby Product Ingredients

- Lavender (also goes by *Lavendula angustifolia*): Okay for mom, but not for baby.
- The paraben class of preservatives: Look for the suffix "-paraben" at the end of ingredient names. The major parabens are methyl-paraben, propylparaben, butylparaben, and ethylparaben.
- Tea tree oil (also goes by *Melaleuca alternifolia*): Also okay for mom but not for baby.
- Soy and its derivatives.
- Chemical sunscreens: Oxybenzone, benzophenone, homosalate, homomethyl, salicylate, 4-methylbenzylidene camphor (4-MBC), parsol, OMC, methoxycinnamate, octinoxate, octyl-dimethyl-PABA, PABA, p-aminobenzoic acid, avobenzone, octyl salicylate, benzyl salicylate, octisalate, octocrylene, ethylhexyl salicylate.
- Dichlorodiphenyltrichloroethane (DDT): This pesticide is no longer used in most of the world.
- Phthalates: Watch for DEHP, DIDP, DINP, BBP, or "fragrance," which may include phthalates not listed in the product ingredients.

Choose to Use: Baby Product Ingredients

- Zinc oxide
- Vitamin E
- Sodium PCA
- Chamomile extract
- Vegetable glycerin
- Calendula oil
- Green tea (*Camellia sinensis*)
- Vanilla bean extract
- Beeswax (*Cera alba*)
- Extra virgin olive oil (*Olea europaea*)
- Castor oil (*Ricinus communis*)

Eczema can be difficult to manage and control. Your pediatrician will guide you in the right direction and tell you when it's time to start using stronger medications like topical steroids.

Baby Sun Protection 101

One of the most common misconceptions when it comes to babies and sunscreen is that you should not apply it to children under the age of six months. In fact, when Melissa was being released from the hospital on a sunny May day after giving birth to her second son, the nurse told her that she should not use sun protection on him. That advice seemed counterintuitive. Every single day we slather sun protection all over our own bodies, which at this point in life is hardly virgin skin. Why would we neglect our newborns, whose delicate skin has never even seen the light of day?

Here's why: "When companies manufacture sunscreen, they have to get FDA approval, as sunscreens are considered drugs because of their active ingredients," explains Dr. Schaffran. "In order to get FDA approval, companies have to go through testing." Six months old is the lower age limit for the human subjects companies are allowed to use in their tests, so when companies do get FDA approval, they can legally recommend sunscreen only for ages six months and above. "But that doesn't mean you can't use it on six months and under. It just means it can't be marketed for babies under six months of age—it's illegal," says Dr. Schaffran.

Another reason doctors don't like to recommend sunscreen on babies under six months is concern about the chemical ingredients. "Many sunscreens have a chemical active ingredient, and those can be very irritating to babies," says Dr. Schaffran. "Especially oxybenzone, which is a chemical with a lot of controversy surrounding it as to whether or not it's safe. The absorption of those chemicals is higher in a baby under six months." Dr. Schaffran recommends the use of mineral-based sunscreens (titanium dioxide and zinc oxide) all the time, with babies six months and under. "They are essentially the same mineral-based ingredients we use in diaper creams," she explains.

In other words, sunscreens for your little ones should essentially have the same ingredients as the sunscreens you used when you were pregnant. Stay away from the chemicals in our "Reduce Your Use" list and use only the minerals titanium dioxide and zinc oxide. Don't worry if the formula goes on a little pasty. We'd rather have our babies be well protected, even if that means looking a little whitewashed.

In applying sunscreen to your baby, make sure you get all the exposed areas thoroughly covered. The best way to fully protect your little one's delicate scalp—even a scalp covered with a full head of hair—is with a sunhat. Another way to protect your baby from the sun is to get baby sunglasses to cover the delicate eye area. We also advise buying an extra sunshade for the stroller; a silver or white one won't absorb the heat and make your baby extra hot. If you're at the beach, keep your baby under the umbrella at all times or invest in a baby outdoor sun tent. We love the PeaPod from Kidco (www.kidco.com).

Pregnant Pause

Ask Dr. Robin Schaffran, Pediatric Dermatologist

We asked Dr. Schaffran pretty much every question under the sun about babies and SPF. Here's what she had to say:

Q: Do we need to slather our children with sunscreen even if we're just taking them outside for a few minutes?

A: I say yes, but the reality is that most people don't—even I don't! Your kids are getting a lot of sun exposure without protection even if you're not intentionally doing it. As a mom, you're never going to be perfect in getting it on all the time, even when you're trying to do your very best. I don't think it's good to be obsessive about anything, but if you're a reasonable person who's trying to do her best in putting sunscreen on her kid, the likelihood is that your child is going to get enough exposure to the sun without sunscreen to make sufficient amounts of vitamin D that it's not going to be an issue.

Q: *Which leads us to the vitamin D issue. What do you say to parents who are worried that their kids aren't getting enough exposure to the sun for optimal vitamin D production?*

A: I don't think you should ever intentionally try to get sun exposure, because unintentionally you're going to get enough—certainly enough to get the vitamin D you need. The risk of sunburn is so much greater in terms of doing damage than the potential benefits of going without sunscreen.

Q: *When is the best time to apply sunscreen to our children? Do we need to do it thirty minutes before leaving the house?*

A: It depends on the sunscreen. For chemical-based sunscreens, the active ingredients require time to penetrate into the skin to do what they're supposed to do. Chemical-based sunscreen ingredients inactivate the ultraviolet rays when they hit the skin. They need to penetrate into the skin in order to have that effect with ultraviolet light, so you need to apply them fifteen to twenty minutes prior to going outside. Mineral-based sunscreens physically block the UV rays, so they don't require penetration and you can apply them right before going outside. But having said that, it's always good to leave yourself a little time before heading out to apply the sunscreen—it's much easier to do it in the house when your kids are not running around or trying to jump in the pool. Plus you'll get a more even application.

Q: *What's the best place and temperature to store sunscreen?*

A: Sunscreen should be stored ideally at room temperature, somewhere between 60 and 85 degrees Fahrenheit. Very high temps can affect the formulation and possibly the effectiveness of the sunscreen.

Q: *What's the shelf life of sunscreen?*

A: Every sunscreen that is on the market should be labeled with an expiration date on the tube. In general, the shelf lives of the mineral-based sunscreens are longer than for chemical sunscreens. The average shelf life for most sunscreens is one to two years from the date of manufacturing. The expiration date is somewhat arbitrary and doesn't necessarily mean the sunscreen is ineffective after that date, but it does mean that the company cannot vouch for its efficacy beyond that time frame.

Q: *How do we know if sunscreen has gone bad?*

A: There is no way to really know if the sunscreen is not effective anymore, other than to put it through expensive laboratory testing. But if the consistency has changed significantly after being in extreme temperatures for a long time, or if it is well past the expiration date, I would advise getting some new sunscreen.

Keep Your Kids Clean—But Not Too Clean

Chances are that your hospital room had a Purell dispenser attached to the wall. Ours did, and you can bet we were dousing our hands in the stuff at the hospital. We didn't want to take any chances exposing our newborns to harmful bacteria. But what about when you get home? Where should you draw the line when it comes to using antibacterial gels for yourself and your kids?

"If your kids are playing in the grass, where there's a lot of potential feces or seriously harmful bacteria, or they go to visit a hospital where there's potential for spreading bacteria or they were around someone who was sick, it's important to use the antibacterial soaps or gels," says Dr. Schaffran. "But soap and water is just fine for regular cleaning. I believe in the germ hypothesis: we're seeing more immune-type diseases in developed countries because kids are not being exposed to enough germs and their immune systems are becoming underdeveloped."

We don't take hand washing lightly and are religious about scrubbing our hands every time we enter the house. We do the same with our kids. And as tempting as it is to douse our kids' hands in an antibacterial gel every time they touch a slobbery toy at someone else's house or a well-intentioned stranger gives them a high-five, we have learned to restrain ourselves and wait until we get to the nearest bathroom to wash their hands with regular old soap (not antibacterial) and water. For those times when we simply cannot wait and are going to be away from home too long, we use an alcohol-free wipe or hand sanitizer. Our friends at BabyGanics created their wipes to be all-around baby cleaners, so we make sure to keep a pack with us at all times to clean their dirty little hands and faces without introducing ingredients that, by killing both good and bad bacteria, might be doing exactly the opposite of what we want them to do.

Baby Steps to a Perfect Bath

We're not going to lie: we both felt like bath time with our babies was a comedy of errors. Add one slippery, crying baby to a tub of water and what you get is a very frustrating yet hilarious experience. Often we would put off bath time for days to avoid the inevitable fiasco.

We had heard from many trusted sources that we didn't actually need to give our babies a bath every day. The common belief is that too much bathing dries out the skin. That turns out not to be true. "Contrary to popular belief, bathing is good for the skin," says Dr. Schaffran. "It hydrates the skin by putting water into the skin." Her advice for keeping babies' skin healthy and moisturized is to soak them in the tub for fifteen to twenty minutes, pat them dry, and apply a good moisturizer within three minutes. So where did the idea that bathing dries out the skin come from? "Bathing can lead to drying out of the skin . . . when there is no moisturizer applied to the skin immediately after the bath to seal in all that hydration," says Dr. Schaffran.

When it comes to bathing your baby, here are the most important points to remember:

- Don't ever leave your baby in the bath by himself! That means ignoring your BlackBerry and any other distractions. Babies can drown in two inches of water, and it takes only a second for an accident to happen.
- Make sure the water is warm, but not as hot as the bathwater you'd like for yourself. Test the water on the inside of your wrist to make sure the temp feels good. We advise setting your hot water heater at no higher than 120 degrees. Twenty-four percent of scald burns for children under the age of four are from hot tap water.
- Make sure the room where you're bathing your baby is at least 75 degrees so that when you take her out she doesn't get cold. Babies lose heat very fast!
- Apply moisturizer immediately after the bath to lock in moisture. The best ingredients to look for in a baby lotion are glycerin and vitamin E.

A Tub We Love

Our favorite tub for newborns is the European-style bucket tub. It may look like a regular old bucket, but it's free of bisphenol A (BPA), polyvinyl chloride (PVC), and phthalates. It also comforts babies by keeping them in the fetal position. The bucket style keeps the water warm for twenty minutes, unlike the standard lie-on-the-back tub, which gets cold fast. For more information, check out the Spa Baby website (www.spababytubs.com).

Clean Water = Happy Baby

Another culprit in the fight against dry skin is water that contains too much chlorine. In fact, chlorine can be a trigger for eczema. It's often added to tap water to kill bacteria, but when it reacts with other elements it can form a toxin called trihalomethanes (THMs), which are linked to a whole host of health issues like asthma and eczema. Our suggestion? Add a water filter to your list of must-buys when your baby is born.

Unhappy with the quality of water in her area, Taslie Skincare founder Tami Main created the Sprite Baby Shower, which filters out chlorine, dirt, and impurities. "If you have a child with sensitive skin or eczema, the filter really helps, as chlorine is very drying to the skin," says Main. After hooking the filter onto your showerhead, you can pull it down and fill up the baby tub. It's great for moms too! "I color my hair, so I use it too," Tami says. You can buy one at www.taslie.com.

Did You Know?

Keeping your baby's skin well moisturized helps prevent dermatitis and eczema.

Talcum Powder: Why You Should Avoid It Like the Plague!

It turns out that talcum powder, the seemingly innocuous substance that's been used on baby's tushies for years, can do major damage to children's lungs. *Time* magazine actually dubbed it the "powder of death."

If that's not enough to scare you away from using it, here's why we recommend not getting the stuff near your baby. The problem with talc is that it's very lightweight and floats into the air without falling down right away. What usually happens is that the talcum powder is sitting next to baby when mom is changing the diaper and the baby grabs the bottle, shakes it, and releases a big cloud of talcum powder. The powder is very irritating to lung tissue. There have been reports of children seriously damaging their lungs after breathing it in.

According to the National Institutes of Health (NIH), accidentally inhaling talcum powder can lead to rapid, shallow breathing, lung failure, and even death. If you still want to powder your little one's behind, use cornstarch—it's a great (and safe) alternative.

The Lowdown on Plastic Packaging

It's not just the contents of baby products that you need to be aware of, but the packaging as well. Some plastic packaging is known to contain xenoestrogens such as bisphenol A (BPA) and di-2-ethylhexyl phthalate (DEHP), chemicals you don't want leaching into your baby's products because of their hormone-disrupting capabilities. You can tell which type of plastic is used in the packaging by looking at the recycle code on the bottom of the bottle—a number with a triangle around it. Try to avoid numbers 7 and 3. Code 3 means the plastic is PVC, which is made with the phthalate DEHP. Not all plastics marked with code 7 are made from polycarbonate, which contains BPA, but unless you know for certain that the plastic packaging of a baby product is BPA-free, be safe and avoid it. Safer choices are plastics with the recycling codes 1, 2, and 4.

Pregnant Pause

Ask Kevin Schwartz and Keith Garber,
Founders of BabyGanics (and Self-Described "Neat Freaks")

Q: *Tell us how BabyGanics was born.*

A: We started with a line of simple household cleaners that were so safe you could drink them and were built so mom and dad could use them liberally and not have any concerns. It developed into personal care, laundry, and hand hygiene. Many doctors and ob-gyns are specifically calling out the fact that moms should not be using any of the toxic chemicals found in the household products we grew up using—basically anything that makes your eyes water.

Q: *What is the common misconception about natural and organic brands?*

A: Just because a product is natural doesn't mean it's safe. People might think that when a product has "coconut-based ingredients," somebody cracked open a coconut, and that somehow cleans things. Obviously that's not exactly how things work. People find out natural and organic products can be irritating, or many times they find that the efficacy has been cut. A solution can get watered down to get it down to a toxicity profile that makes it safer, but now you lose the efficacy.

Q: *So, as parents, how can we trust that a product is indeed safe?*

A: The birth of a new child is a tipping point in life when you start to do better for yourself and your new child, better than you've ever done before. Find brands you can trust. Generally brands have standards going across a lot of different products and platforms. The folks that are doing it right have one straight set of standards across the solutions and products they offer. Find those and go deep within a brand. It's very rare that you'll see a huge contradiction between two products within the same brand. Find brands you trust and partner with them as a consumer.

Q: *What's the story on your baby wipes? They absolutely rock!*

A: You don't find that thickness anywhere. The market is going toward this subtle thinning of wipes. As you see the price at the pump going up, the price of raw materials skyrockets too. There are subtleties that some consumers don't necessarily see. On the household side, it's slight reductions in active ingredients. On the baby wipes side, it's the thinning of the thickness. With our fragrance-free wipes, we wanted to have a minimalistic formulation that had enough cleaning properties to really work, but no additives and no fragrance on a really luxurious wipe. There was recently a study on what percentage of baby wipes is actually used for the tush versus the hands and face, and it was a huge percentage, like 50 percent. So a lightbulb went off for a lot of companies, and they thought, "We can have another product out there." But we combined that in one product. Our goal was for this to be an all-in-one wipe.

Q: *What ingredients are on your "do not use" list?*

A: The big things to avoid are the hormone-disrupting chemicals. Those are the chemicals found in baby's bloodstream at birth passed on through mom. If we were all to go get our blood tested right now, we'd find chemicals that have been banned for upwards of twenty years, passed on from our parents and their parents. They're persistent chemicals that will in fact never go away. The problem is that new chemicals are being introduced into the environment at a faster rate than the old ones are being identified and banned. Realistically, the only way it's going to change is with a greater level of education and an increased demand from the consumer. The policy needs to change from "innocent until proven guilty" to "guilty until proven innocent" when it comes to chemicals in products used in our homes and around our families.

Q: *Both of you are dads to two young kids. How's that "neat freak" thing working out?*

A: We don't think you can live as a neat freak and have smiles on little faces at the same time.

Baby-Smart Product Picks

Shampoo and Body Wash

When shopping for a baby cleanser, it's important to stay away from products containing harsh sulfates, which could irritate baby's skin. Another accessory you'll want for bath time is a soft, thin washcloth to help you get to all of your baby's crevices.

- BabyGanics Foamin' Fun Newborn Bodywash and Shampoo (fragrance-free)
- Lavanila Healthy Baby Wash
- Babo Botanicals Oatmilk Calendula Moisturizing Baby Shampoo and Wash
- Taslie Head to Toe Body Wash
- Exederm Baby Eczema Wash
- Belli Baby Calm Me Hair and Body Wash

Diaper Cream

Diaper creams serve an important function in baby care. They create a barrier between your baby's sensitive skin and moisture inside the diaper, which is the main cause of diaper rash. Look for diaper creams with zinc oxide, an effective and long-lasting physical barrier that has been around for ages and has few safety concerns attached to it.

- Lavanila: The Healthy Baby Bottom
- Method Baby Squeaky Green Diaper Cream
- BabyGanics Hiney Helper Diaper Cream

Wipes

We use baby wipes on everything from baby's bum to our own hands. We never leave the house without a pack tucked away in our bags. Since wipes need to be kept moist, we suggest keeping the package in a large plastic bag to ensure they don't get exposed to air. Our favorite picks are all free of the bad stuff and great at keeping us and our babies clean.

- BabyGanics Thick N' Kleen Wipes
- Pampers Sensitive Wipes

- Earth's Best TenderCare Chlorine-Free Wipes
- Natracare Organic Baby Wipes

Sunblock

All of our sunblock picks are free of xenoestrogens and made instead with the minerals zinc oxide and titanium dioxide. The mineral blocks sometimes leave a white film, but we're okay with that as long as we know our kids are getting protection the safe way.

- Episencial Sunny Sunscreen SPF 35
- Lavanila Healthy Baby Block SPF 40
- Dr. Robin for Kids All Natural Chemical-Free Sunscreen SPF 30+
- Babo Botanicals Invisible Sun Stick

Lotion

- Belli Baby Nourish Me Enriched Body Lotion
- Exederm Hydrating Baby Lotion
- Babo Botanicals Oatmilk Calendula Moisturizing Baby Lotion
- Taslie Moisturizing Lotion

Being a Baby-Smart Mom

Bringing our firstborns home from the hospital might very well have been the most terrifying moment of our lives. We second-guessed everything we did. Should we let the swing rock him to sleep? How long should we let him cry? Did he get enough to eat?

It's completely normal for first-time moms to feel uneasy and to make mistakes. It's also typical to turn to others for help with decision-making. But before you just start using the same brand of wipes or baby lotion that your mom or your best friend used for their babies, it's important to do your own research. New studies come out every day. We suggest staying on top of the news by signing up for Google alerts that contain key words such as "baby skin care," "baby safety," and "baby health."

Taking the smart route is often not the easiest route to take. We know how tempting it is just to buy the sunscreen or the baby lotion that's easiest to find. We also know how much simpler it would be not to have to look at any labels at all. But introducing potential health issues like the ones associated with the ingredients we're warning you about is not a chance worth taking where our children are involved.

Becoming a mother transforms you into the CEO of your family, so it's up to you to do the legwork for your kids and be your own ingredient police. No one is going to do it for you, not even the government. We urge you to start speaking up and to call your favorite brands to ask them about their ingredients. As mothers, we have tremendous buying power (in the United States we influence over 85 percent of household purchases, which totals about $2.1 trillion!), and we *can* change how things are done. Let this be the start of a revolution to make the world a safer place for our children.

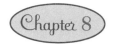
Mom- and Baby-Smart Product Shopping Guide

The chapters of this book have listed the relevant products that screened at least 90 percent free of suspected teratogens. The products marked with a ♥ screened completely free of teratogens during our screening process. Here we provide a complete list of pregnancy and baby-smart product picks and information on why they're our favorites and where to find them.

Mom-Smart Products

Face Cleansers

bareMinerals Skincare Purifying Cleanser

Why we love it: This cleanser is made with a proprietary blend called RareMinerals ActiveSoil Complex. Just the name sounds like it's going to do something spectacular for your skin—and it does! This new generation of minerals speeds up cell turnover. Translation? It helps bring the fresher skin underneath to the surface, subsequently ridding your skin of blemishes, discolorations, and dry skin.

Where to buy it: Bare Escentuals (www.bareescentuals.com)

Belli Acne Cleansing Facial Wash ♥

Why we love it: The key ingredient in Belli's best-selling acne cleanser is pregnancy-friendly lactic acid, which gently cleanses and exfoliates breakout-prone skin. We both used this product religiously during our pregnancies and loved the fact that our skin remained clear for those nine months. This skin saver also contains antioxidant-rich green tea and cucumber extracts to fight the signs of aging, as well as lemon peel oil to brighten skin.

Where to buy it: Belli (www.belliskincare.com)

Burt's Bees Radiance Daily Cleanser

Why we love it: This is a milky, lotion-based cleanser, which is an excellent formula for those of us no longer in our twenties (ahem). We're also big fans of the jojoba beads and fruit acid that gently exfoliate the skin, leaving it brighter, hence the name. The royal jelly in here, made from honeybees, is a nourishing natural ingredient packed with vitamins and minerals.

Where to buy it: Burt's Bees (www.burtsbees.com)

Duchess Marden Damascena Crème Cleanser

Why we love it: This creamy, sophisticated cleanser is an elegant answer for skin that's graduated from foamy bubbles. Made with healing and hydrating rose oil and housed in a gorgeous glass bottle, this collagen-building cleanser is truly a luxury product!

Where to buy it: saffronrouge (www.saffronrouge.com)

Goldfaden Daily Cleanser ♥

Why we love it: The entire Goldfaden line uses red tea, which has fifty times the antioxidant power of green tea (who knew!). Celebrity dermatologist Dr. Gary Goldfaden combines advanced medical high tech with natural botanicals to create all his products.

The Daily Cleanser gently removes makeup while purifying the complexion.

Where to buy it: Goldfaden Skincare (www.goldfaden.com)

Intelligent Nutrients Anti-Aging Cleanser ♥

Why we love it: The man behind Intelligent Nutrients is Horst Rechelbacher, an eco-mastermind and the original founder of Aveda. He grows all the plant ingredients for Intelligent Nutrients skin care products on his organic farm in Wisconsin. This non-foaming, lotion-based cleanser feels like luxury on the skin, while the food-grade, plant-based ingredients leave the face feeling insanely soft and hydrated.

Where to buy it: Intelligent Nutrients
(www.intelligentnutrients.com)

Neutrogena Naturals Fresh Cleansing Makeup Remover

Why we love it: Many brands have jumped on the "natural" bandwagon but continue to use less-than-healthy ingredients. Not so with Neutrogena, which tapped into a team of experts with scientific and integrative health backgrounds to produce this line. The result? Effective and eco-friendly products free of harsh chemicals like sulfates, dyes, and parabens. This cleanser does an amazing job of removing makeup and passed our clean washcloth test: it left no trace of makeup on our white towel after use.

Where to buy it: Neutrogena Naturals
(naturals.neutrogena.com)

Ole Henriksen African Red Tea Foaming Cleanser

Why we love it: This award-winning cleanser (it was named "Best Natural Cleanser" at the Natural Health Beauty Awards in 2009) is packed with vitamin C and the age-fighting antioxidant African red tea. We love the gentle foaming formula that doesn't strip the skin of moisture but does an amazing job of getting rid of dirt and makeup. Another plus is the bright scent, courtesy of grapefruit, tangerine, and orange extracts.

Where to buy it: Ole Henriksen (www.olehenriksen.com)

Origins Checks and Balances Frothy Face Wash

Why we love it: A little goes a long way with this skin-smart cleanser. The broadleaf kelp extract keeps excess oil in check, while wheat protein balances out dry areas (hence the name!). The gentle formula also includes tourmaline, which is said to make water "wetter" so that it rids the skin of more dirt and sebum.

Where to buy it: Origins (www.origins.com)

The Organic Pharmacy Tea Tree Oil and Peppermint Face Wash

Why we love it: Made with some of our favorite pregnancy-approved acne cleansing ingredients, this is one antibacterial wash that even those with ultra-sensitive skin can feel comfortable using. Plus, the peppermint is the perfect morning pick-me-up!

Where to buy it: The Organic Pharmacy
(www.theorganicpharmacy.com)

Tata Harper Regenerating Cleanser

Why we love it: We have a girl crush on Tata Harper, a mom herself. Tata formulates all the products in her skin care line on her Vermont farm, sourcing ingredients from the clay soil of Lake Champlain as well as from farms as far-flung as the Amazon, Israel, and New Zealand. Using this cleanser gives us a little taste of her organic farming lifestyle. It's loaded with essential oils and antioxidants that hydrate while balancing out sebum production (so helpful during pregnancy!).

Where to buy it: Tata Harper Skincare
(www.tataharperskincare.com)

Eye Cream

Belli Eye Brightening Cream ♥
Why we love it: It instantly cools and refreshes tired eyes on contact and comes with an added bonus—vitamin K, which helps combat dark under-eye circles.

Where to buy it: Belli (www.belliskincare.com)

Naturopathica Primrose Eye and Lip Cream
Why we love it: We love double-duty products, and this one treats two areas that are the first to show fine lines—the eyes and the upper lip. It's made with evening primrose oil to improve the skin's elasticity and acai fruit oil to regenerate it.

Where to buy it: Naturopathica (www.naturopathica.com)

REN Active 7 Radiant Eye Gel
Why we love it: Like an eye lift in a bottle, this cooling, firming gel will really help you look more awake. Think of it as a pregnancy-smart cosmetic alternative to your morning coffee!

Where to buy it: REN Clean Skincare (www.renskincare.com)

ShiKai Borage Dry Skin Therapy Eye Cream
Why we love it: This ultra-rich eye cream comforts the driest skin and gives the eye area a luminous appearance. We love dotting it on after we apply our makeup for a little glow!

Where to buy it: ShiKai (www.shikai.com)

Weleda Wild Rose Smoothing Eye Cream
Why we love it: We know how puffy you can get during pregnancy! This fragrance-free eye cream uses rosehip seed oil to battle puffiness.
Where to buy it: Drugstore.com (www.drugstore.com)

Yes To Blueberries Firming Eye Cream
Why we love it: Blueberries are our favorite super-food. They're loaded with antioxidants, so imagine the benefits of using them in skin care, especially around the eye area. We've been using this eye cream for months and can attest to its firming power.
Where to buy it: Yes To Carrots (www.yestocarrots.com)

Lip Care

EOS Lip Sphere in Peppermint ♥
Why we love it: This funky-looking balm is not your average lip product. Sure, the mod sphere is fun to use, but it's all about the balm itself, which is made with lip-smoothing shea butter and jojoba oil. The tingly peppermint oil is like a breath mint for your lips.
Where to buy it: eos (www.evolutionofsmooth.com)

Hurraw Moon Balm
Why we love it: A lip balm made specifically for nighttime is pretty genius in our book. That's when our lips need a big injection of moisture the most. This super-creamy formula is made with extremely nourishing ingredients, including avocado oil, argan oil, and rosehip seed oil. The balm also has chamomile to give your lips the equivalent of a calming cup of nighttime tea.
Where to buy it: Hurraw! (www.hurrawbalm.com)

Intelligent Nutrients Certified Organic Lip Delivery Nutrition
Why we love it: Made with Intelligent Nutrients' special blend of antioxidants and other nutritious ingredients, this balm is one you won't have to worry about ingesting, as inevitably you will. We also love the generous size—ours lasted a lonnng time!
  Where to buy it: Intelligent Nutrients
      (www.intelligentnutrients.com)

Weleda Everon Lip Balm
Why we love it: The lovely rose and vanilla scent is addicting—and comes from all-natural essential oils. Beeswax and shea butter nip dryness in the bud, while the healing and antiseptic properties of rose wax treat cracked and chapped lips.
  Where to buy it: Weleda (www.usa.weleda.com)

Face Moisturizers

Aesop Fabulous Face Oil
Why we love it: We were always trained to think that oil is bad for your complexion. But it turns out that the right kind of oil is actually really good for your skin—especially as we approach our forties. We're hooked on this amazing-smelling blend of floral extracts that leaves the face glowing and hydrated without even a trace of grease left over. Another thing that makes this oil truly fabulous is that it's completely free of preservatives, thanks to its water-free formula. The bottle is smartly made with UV-blocking amber to keep the ingredients stable.
  Where to buy it: Aesop (www.aesop.com)

Belli Healthy Glow Facial Hydrator ♥
Why we love it: This new addition to the Belli lineup is loaded with skin-smart ingredients such as vitamin C and grapeseed oil (for

glowing skin) and chamomile (to soothe irritated skin). It's hard to find a lightweight moisturizer that really hydrates, but this one does the trick! We use it day and night.

Where to buy it: Belli (www.belliskincare.com)

Egyptian Magic ♥

Why we love it: There's a reason why celebrities and beauty insiders are obsessed with this all-purpose skin cream. After rubbing the balm in our hands, which turned it into a light oil, we applied it to some dry patches on our faces and necks, and they immediately felt softer. Models use this cream after photo shoots and fashion shows to heal the skin—and now we're hooked too.

Where to buy it: Egyptian Magic (www.egyptianmagic.com)

Embryolisse Emulsion for Dry Skin

Why we love it: Embryolisse is a French company whose products are reaching cult status in the United States. This luxurious-feeling moisturizing cream literally melts into the skin, leaving behind a slight dewy sheen.

Where to buy it: Embryolisse (www.embryolisseusa.com)

Intelligent Nutrients Certified Organic Anti-Aging Moisture

Why we love it: This hydrator is the match for Intelligent Nutrients' stellar Anti-Aging Cleanser. It goes on super-light and is packed with good-for-your-skin ingredients that make skin baby-soft. We also love the natural scent, which is a lovely combination of the fragrant essential oils inside.

Where to buy it: Intelligent Nutrients (www.intelligentnutrients.com)

Jurlique Herbal Recovery Night Cream
Why we love it: Loaded with eight herbs and flowers, this amazing-smelling night cream is formulated without any synthetic fragrances. Even though it's a night cream, it goes on very lightly, and our faces still felt soft and hydrated the next morning.
Where to buy it: Jurlique (www.jurlique.com)

Kate Somerville Oil-Free Moisturizer
Why we love it: This is a great choice for those who have breakouts yet still want a moisturizer loaded with benefits. The oil-free formula is ideal for sensitive and acne-prone skin, while the sea plant extracts inside encourage collagen production and help tone the skin. We also love the mattifying effect of this moisturizer.
Where to buy it: Kate Somerville Skin Health Experts
(www.katesomerville.com)

Korres Quercetin & Oak Anti-Wrinkle Night Cream
Why we love it: Now that we're not in our twenties anymore, we need our moisturizers to deeply hydrate and fight wrinkles and fine lines. This moisturizer does all of that. When you're expecting, it's important to lay off all the heavy-duty anti-aging treatments, and this top-selling night cream, which is free of parabens, is a great choice.
Where to buy it: Korres (www.korresusa.com)

Shampoo

Burt's Bees Super Shiny Grapefruit and Sugar Beet Shampoo
Why we love it: Like a delicious salad for our hair, this offbeat combination of citrus oils and sugar beets is a recipe for boosting the shine factor.
Where to buy it: Burt's Bees (www.burtsbees.com)

Moroccan Oil Moisture Repair Shampoo
Why we love it: This is one of the only shampoos that we would use on a daily basis. Argan oil is the secret weapon, mixed with vitamins to shield hair from the environment.
    Where to buy it: MoroccanOil (www.moroccanoil.com)

Conditioner

Know! Conditioner
Why we love it: Created by two seasoned celebrity hairstylists, this new hair care brand is getting a lot of attention from the media for its clean formulations. The color-safe conditioner has quickly become a favorite of ours. It just goes to show that you don't need a whole host of nasty synthetics to get your hair looking its best.
    Where to buy it: Know! Hair & Body
          (www.knowhairandbody.com)

Peter Lamas Soy Hydrating Conditioner ♥
Why we love it: We were thrilled that this deeply moisturizing conditioner completely passed teratology screening. Made with protein-rich soy and a host of vitamins and botanicals, it left our color-treated hair incredibly soft and frizz-free.
    Where to buy it: Peter Lamas (www.peterlamas.com)

Hairstyling Products

Couture Colour Pequi Oil Treatment
Why we love it: A favorite of some top Hollywood hairstylists, this hair-smoothing treatment is made from the pequi fruit, found in the Amazon rain forest. A little drop tames the frizzies after a blowdry.
    Where to buy it: Couture Colour (www.couturecolour.com)

Josie Maran Argan Oil Hair Serum
Why we love it: Is there anything argan oil can't do? This wonder
oil also helps seal split ends and gives the hair a nice shine.
　Where to buy it: Josie Maran Cosmetics
　　　　　(www.josiemarancosmetics.com)

Sunblock: Face

Belli Anti-Chloasma Facial Sunscreen SPF 25 ♥
Why we love it: This is Melissa's desert island beauty product. It's
the ultimate multitasking product—sunscreen, moisturizer, and
skin tint in one. Made with mineral sunscreens and a tint that magically matches almost all skin tones, this teratogen-free sunscreen
is the must-have product in the beauty wardrobe of every woman—
pregnant or not. We use it every single day under makeup or instead of it.
　Where to buy it: Belli (www.belliskincare.com)

Josie Maran Argan Oil Daily Moisturizer with SPF 40+
Why we love it: Josie's secret ingredient is argan oil, a synthetic-
free, vitamin-rich oil that repairs and reverses sun damage and im-
proves skin tone and clarity. This ultra-lightweight sunblock is
fast-absorbing and incredibly gentle—it's great for sensitive skin. It
also works as an amazing makeup primer.
　Where to buy it: Josie Maran Cosmetics
　　　　　(www.josiemarancosmetics.com)

Super by Perricone Daylight Savings SPF 25 Moisturizer
Why we love it: If there's one thing Dr. Perricone knows about, it's
super-foods—the antioxidant-loaded foods that make skin look
young and beautiful. His line of skin care, Super, features the

molecules found in many of his beloved super-foods. This multi-tasking daily mineral-sunscreen-and-moisturizer-in-one uses the antioxidant turmeric to deliver UV protection along with a nice glow and a hint of shimmer from the minerals.

Where to buy it: Super by Dr. Nicholas Perricone
(www.getsuper.com)

Sunblock: Body

Aubrey Natural Sun SPF 30+

Why we love it: This sunblock has an incredible smooth texture that rubs in seamlessly and leaves a gorgeous shine to the skin. It's a beach bag must-have!

Where to buy it: Aubrey Organics
(www.aubrey-organics.com)

Josie Maran Argan Sun Protection for Body 30+

Why we love it: Whatever the time of year, we don't like to take any chances with sun exposure. This daily wear sunblock features Josie's awesome argan oil, which means it also repairs skin and helps fight Father Time.

Where to buy it: Josie Maran Cosmetics
(www.josiemarancosmetics.com)

Marie Veronique Organics Kid Safe Screen

Why we love it: Not all kid-safe sunscreens scored highly in our teratology screening process, but this one did! We love its antioxidant-rich, non-nano zinc oxide formula because it blends in without leaving any white behind—a tough feat!

Where to buy it: Marie Veronique Organics
(www.mvorganics.com)

Soap and Body Wash

100 Percent Pure Organic Virgin Coconut Body Wash
Why we love it: We literally feel like we've taken a tropical island vacation every time we lather up with this heavenly scented coconut body wash. Thanks to the super-clean vegan ingredients and the generous size, this body wash is one of our favorite new products.
Where to buy it: 100% Pure (www.100percentpure.com)

Belli Pampered Pregnancy Body Wash ♥
Why we love it: Both of us had dry, itchy skin during pregnancy. Belli's body wash was our go-to daily body cleanser. It gently yet thoroughly cleanses without making your skin feel two sizes too small.
Where to buy it: Belli (www.belliskincare.com)

Dove Sensitive Skin Beauty Bar
Why we love it: We were thrilled when this bar soap from a brand we grew up with scored highly in teratology screening. It's fragrance-free and gentle enough for sensitive skin types. The moisturizing formula won't dry out your hands—which is important if you're a vigilant hand washer like us.
Where to buy it: Drugstore.com (www.drugstore.com)

Kiss My Face Olive Oil Bar Soap, Pure Olive Oil ♥
Why we love it: This gigantic slab of soap gets you as clean as you're going to get—literally. The completely pregnancy-friendly formula has only three ingredients—olive oil, water, and sodium chloride. You won't find any artificial colors or fragrances, but what you *will* find is one big, pure bar of good soap.
Where to buy it: Kiss My Face (www.kissmyface.com)

Whole Foods Market Organic Castile Peppermint Soap
Why we love it: You won't find a more versatile soap than this minty fresh liquid. Though we use it in the shower for our whole bodies, you can use it to clean everything from your pets to your kids. The organic peppermint oil leaves behind an energizing tingly sensation.
Where to buy it: Whole Foods stores

Yes To Cucumbers Calming Shower Gel
Why we love it: Cucumber is one of our favorite soothing ingredients, and we love how it makes our skin feel cool and refreshed, especially first thing in the morning. Green tea and Dead Sea minerals are also in the mix of this generously sized bottle of shower gel. We also use this instead of shaving cream!
Where to buy it: Yes To Carrots (www.yestocarrots.com)

Body Lotions and Stretch Mark Creams

100 Percent Pure Organic French Lavender Body Cream
Why we love it: Fruit oils along with cocoa and avocado butters do an amazing job of hydrating and softening the skin. We love the light lavender scent, which is from essential oils, not synthetic fragrances. Be sure to use this one only on yourself, since lavender is not recommended for use on babies.
Where to buy it: 100% Pure (www.100percentpure.com)

Belli All Day Moisture Body Lotion♥
Why we love it: We're addicted (and we've heard we're not alone) to Belli's All Day Moisture Body Lotion. It's designed for the driest skin types and features the fresh uplifting essence of lemon.
Where to buy it: Belli (www.belliskincare.com)

Belli Elasticity Oil ♥
Why we love it: This beloved oil is recommended by ob-gyns all over the country because its ingredients have been well researched and it helps to maintain the look of healthy skin while the skin is rapidly stretching. It's also used in five-star spas for prenatal massage. We loved slathering it over our tummies during pregnancy— it was a ritual we looked forward to. We imagined the baby inside our belly getting a little massage from it too.
Where to buy it: Belli (www.belliskincare.com)

Belli Stretch Mark Minimizing Cream ♥
Why we love it: After the stretching was done, we relied on this amazing cream to help fade the marks left behind. It's made with darutoside and registril—botanical ingredients that have been scientifically reported to reduce the appearance of a stretch mark's length (by up to 52 percent) and depth (by up to 72 percent).
Where to buy it: Belli (www.belliskincare.com)

California Baby Natural Pregnancy Emulsion
Why we love it: Light and rich, this approved-for-pregnancy lotion is awesome at moisturizing the itchy skin on the growing belly. We also love the delicate scent, courtesy of Roman chamomile, lemon, and peppermint essential oils.
Where to buy it: California Baby (www.californiababy.com)

Erbaviva Stretch Mark Cream ♥
Why we love it: From one of our favorite mama brands, this cream is packed with beneficial essential oils as well as shea butter. It glides right into skin and leaves no greasy residue.
Where to buy it: Erbaviva (www.erbaviva.com)

Terralina Fragrance Free Body Lotion ♥
Why we love it: There are no false claims on this bottle. A no-nonsense, good-for-your-skin lotion packed with soothing ingredients like shea butter, olive oil, jojoba, and barley, it will literally melt into your skin.
   Where to buy it: Terralina (www.terralina.com)

Deodorant

Lavanila: The Healthy Deodorant
Why we love it: Made with a beta glucan technology, this soothing, good-looking deodorant really works! We're hooked on the vanilla coconut scent.
   Where to buy it: Lavanila (www.lavanila.com)

Tom's of Maine Long-Lasting Natural
Aluminum-Free Deodorant
Why we love it: The mineral zinc is the secret ingredient in this odor-absorbing deodorant stick. Zinc ricinoleate, as it turns out, traps odor molecules and absorbs nasty odors.
   Where to buy it: Tom's of Maine (www.tomsofmaine.com)

Makeup: Concealer

Amazing Cosmetics Amazing Concealer
Why we love it: It's no wonder this creamy concealer has won top honors from beauty editors. Though it may be pricier than others on the market, a little goes a long way. Just one teeny dot is enough to cover an entire under-eye area.
   Where to buy it: Amazing Cosmetics
      (www.amazingcosmetics.com)

Boots No. 7 Quick Cover Blemish Stick
Why we love it: This portable, diaper-friendly stick covers every imperfection under the sun, not to mention sun spots! Thanks to zinc oxide, the easy-to-blend formula also fights shine and helps to control oil.
>*Where to buy it:* Drugstore.com (www.drugstore.com)

Christopher Drummond Duo Phase Concealer
Why we love it: We are huge fans of multitasking products, so this one gets our top vote in that department. With a silky texture that works just as well under the eyes as it does on top of blemishes, this concealer can even be used as a light foundation. Drummond, a former model, uses only strong essential oils as preservatives.
>*Where to buy it:* Christopher Drummond Beauty
>(www.christopherdrummond.com)

Vapour Illusionist Concealer
Why we love it: This is one of the brands we fell hard for during the writing of this book. After trying this beautiful concealer—it literally melted into our skin—we were left wondering why any company uses harmful chemicals in their products when nontoxic ingredients can feel this good on the skin.
>*Where to buy it:* Vapour Organic Beauty
>(www.vapourbeauty.com)

Makeup: Foundation
Alima Pure Satin Matte Foundation ♥
Why we love it: Alima is a new brand of products made with pure minerals and no fillers. Using a loose mineral powder instead of the typical liquid foundation does take some getting used to, but this

makeup artist–created brand—with over sixty shades of foundation—makes it well worth it.

Where to buy it: Alima Pure (www.alimapure.com)

bareMinerals SPF 15 Foundation ♥
Why we love it: This foundation makes our complexion look peaches-and-creamy with minimal effort. bareMinerals was our first introduction to mineral makeup, and we still think of it as one of the best.

Where to buy it: Bare Escentuals (www.bareescentuals.com)

Dr.Hauschka Translucent Makeup
Why we love it: When we want that effortless look, we turn to this tinted moisturizer-foundation hybrid. It truly looks like your own skin when it comes out of the tube, and it blends in seamlessly. It's perfect for smearing on before a playdate or a morning pre-school run.

Where to buy it: Dr.Hauschka Cosmetics
(www.dr.hauschka.com)

INIKA Liquid Mineral Foundation
Why we love it: We do love our mineral makeups, but sometimes we prefer the manageability of a liquid formula, which is why we love this foundation that marries the two. It's filled with antioxidants to protect and moisturizing ingredients to soothe.

Where to buy it: saffronrouge (www.saffronrouge.com)

Jane Iredale Amazing Base SPF 20
Why we love it: Recommended by the Skin Cancer Foundation for its great sun protection, this lightweight mineral powder founda-

tion is gentle enough for women who suffer from skin care issues like rosacea and eczema. Another plus? It's a fabulous summertime option because it's waterproof!

Where to buy it: Jane Iredale (shop.janeiredale.com)

Living Nature Illuminating Tint ♥

Why we love it: From New Zealand's top natural skin care brand comes a must-have product we have fallen for. A little lighter than a foundation, but with more coverage than a tinted moisturizer, this may just be the best compromise between the two we've ever tried. It leaves the skin with a crazy gorgeous glow.

Where to buy it: saffronrouge (www.saffronrouge.com)

Maybelline Mineral Power Powder Foundation

Why we love it: We were psyched to learn that one of our best-loved drugstore brands came out with a pregnancy-smart foundation, and it's great! The pure minerals, which contain no fragrances or preservatives, smooth the skin and reduce redness.

Where to buy it: Maybelline (www.maybelline.com)

Vapour Atmosphere Luminous Foundation

Why we love it: This creamy foundation literally makes our skin glow and our pores disappear—genius! Made with mineral pigments and natural vitamins, the products are extra gentle for sensitive skin. One of the founders is the former president of Kevyn Aucoin, so it's no wonder the makeup is professional quality and super-easy to use.

Where to buy it: Vapour Organic Beauty
(www.vapourbeauty.com)

W3LL People Universalist
Why we love it: This multipurpose stick—you can use it on lids, lips, cheeks, bridge of the nose—adds a pop of color or a gleam of sheen to accent areas. It comes in nudes and pinks and has won a valuable spot in our diaper bags!
Where to buy it: W3LL People (www.w3llpeople.com)

Makeup: Tinted Moisturizer

Living Nature Tinted Moisturizer ♥
Why we love it: We've been searching for a tinted moisturizer that also gets rid of shiny areas, and we found it! Yet another awesome product from Living Nature, this moisturizer leaves behind a matte finish while covering redness and splotches and letting your skin shine through.
Where to buy it: saffronrouge (www.saffronrouge.com)

Makeup: Powder

Koh Gen Do Natural Lighting Powder ♥
Why we love it: Movie and TV makeup artists are cult followers of Koh Gen Do. All its products are made with the specific needs of TV and movie stars in mind. High-definition is incredibly unforgiving, but this light beige powder, which uses ultra-fine pearl powder, magically diffuses light to make skin look utterly flawless.
Where to buy it: Koh Gen Do (www.kohgendo.com)

Makeup: Blush and Bronzer

Josie Maran Argan Cream Blush
Why we love it: We love cream formulations for blush—they leave the skin looking a little younger and fresher, in our opinion. Dab a bit of Sunrise (a sheer pink) high on the cheekbones and you'll look like a happy, glowing mama.

Where to buy it: Josie Maran Cosmetics
(www.josiemarancosmetics.com)

Josie Maran Argan Bronzing Powder

Why we love it: This powder is universally flattering and build-able—meaning that you can look anywhere from just a touch bronze to full-on sun-worshiper.
Where to buy it: Josie Maran Cosmetics
(www.josiemarancosmetics.com)

Tarte Mineral Powder Bronzer

Why we love it: When we crave that beachy goddess look in the dead of winter, we turn to this shimmery bronzing powder. The pressed minerals leave less mess than the loose kind, so this is the perfect bronzer to use on the go. Our favorite shade is Park Avenue Princess.
Where to buy it: Tarte (www.tartecosmetics.com)

W3LL People Hedonist Luminous Mineral Bronzer ♥

Why we love it: This bronzer leaves skin with a soft luminescent dusting of golden goodness! In the summer, we love it for all over—neck, décolletage, shoulders.
Where to buy it: W3LL People (www.w3llpeople.com)

Makeup: Eyes

Urban Decay 24/7 Glide-On Shadow Pencil in Sin

Why we love it: This product is an eye liner, it's an eye shadow—it's both! We were thrilled to discover this handy eye shadow pencil that leaves lids washed with a cool color. The pliable formula makes it super-easy to smudge, line, and shade. We think Sin, a beautiful neutral champagne hue, is a yummy mummy essential.
Where to buy it: Urban Decay Cosmetics (www.urbandecay.com)

Kjaer Weis Eye Shadow

Why we love it: Each Kjaer Weis product comes in a gorgeous re-fillable silver compact. We love the long-lasting pearlized finish of her eye shadows. The neutral shades are a working mom's dream.

Where to buy it: Kjaer Weis (www.kjaerweis.com)

INIKA Eyeliner

Why we love it: Made with sustainable palm oil, these liners have a rich and creamy texture that would make any big-time makeup company green with envy. Each liner comes with a built-in sharp-ener on the lid—genius! We love Sapphire—a midnight blue that makes eyes look insanely vibrant.

Where to buy it: saffronrouge (www.saffronrouge.com)

INIKA Mineral Eye Shadow

Why we love it: The pigments in these mineral eye shadows are amaz-ing. The little pots are packed with colors from soft pink and platinum to turquoise. You can use these colors anywhere on the face too.

Where to buy it: saffronrouge (www.saffronrouge.com)

Gabriel Cosmetics Eye Liner

Why we love it: Founder Gabriel DeSantino has developed a color palette with beautiful shades that all women can wear. His kohl eyeliner glides on seamlessly and doesn't pull at the eyes when ap-plied. We think his charcoal is a date night must.

Where to buy it: Gabriel Cosmetics, Inc.
(www.gabrielcosmeticsinc.com)

Lavera Volumizing Mascara

Why we love it: Finding a good mascara that could stand up to our screening wasn't easy. Luckily, we found Lavera. This paraben-free tube of beauty editor–loved mascara uses jojoba and wild rose oils to add volume, length, and definition.

Where to buy it: Lavera Naturkosmetik (www.lavera.com)

Makeup: Lips

Intelligent Nutrients Lip Delivery Antioxidant Gloss in Purple Maze

Why we love it: We are in awe of just about every product from Intelligent Nutrients, and this cool-colored lip gloss is no exception. It leaves the lips with a kiss of pretty berry shade and a wonderfully soft finish. One of our biggest grievances with most lip glosses is being too glossy—they attract everything from strands of hair to potato chip crumbs. Not so with this one. We'll even kiss our little munchkins with the stuff slathered on.

Where to buy it: Intelligent Nutrients

(www.intelligentnutrients.com)

Zuzu Luxe Lip Liner in Innocence

Why we love it: We searched long and hard for a perfect neutral lip liner to recommend in this book, and we're so thrilled to have found one! This lip liner defines the lips and creates the perfect foundation to help lip glosses and lipsticks stay put.

Where to buy it: Gabriel Cosmetics, Inc.

(www.gabrielcosmeticsinc.com)

Nail Polish

Butter London

Why we love it: We are obsessed with this nontoxic (it's free of formaldehyde, toluene, phthalates, and parabens), fashion-forward line of lacquers. At the helm is the magnificently cool British style maven Nonie Crème. Yummy Mummy—a taupey-beige that looks good on literally everyone—is our go-to manicure shade and makes us feel like yummy mummies indeed.

Where to buy it: Butter London (www.butterlondon.com)

Essie
Why we love it: Essie Weingarten, a brilliant businesswoman and very chic lady, made her brand 3-Free, and we couldn't be happier. Her shades are always on trend, and the formulas wear exceptionally well.

Where to buy it: Essie (www.essie.com)

Lippmann Collection
Why we love it: Deborah Lippmann is the celebrity manicurist behind this line of ultra-cool colors. Her genius colors often come from collaborations with fashion designers and celebrities. Lippmann Collection is always a presence backstage at runway shows and on fashion shoots.

Where to buy it: Deborah Lippmann
(www.lippmanncollection.com)

NARS
Why we love it: The strikingly beautiful shades in the NARS collection are all 3-Free. Get a pre-baby pedicure with the shocking pink Schiap. A bright and perfect pedicure makes the whole hospital experience feel a little more glamorous.

Where to buy it: NARS (www.narscosmetics.com)

Revlon
Why we love it: We were thrilled to learn that Revlon, one of our favorite drugstore brands, went 3-Free. The colors in this line are literally limitless!

Where to buy it: Revlon Cosmetics (www.revlon.com)

RGB
Why we love it: In the world of nail polish, RGB has got to be one of the chicest brands around. Its gorgeous selection of rich, neutral colors is a favorite of the fashion and celebrity crowd.
Where to buy it: RGB (www.rgbcosmetics.com)

Zoya
Why we love it: From creamy nude shades to mod mattes and fun metallics, there's something for everyone in Zoya's range of over three hundred colors. Founded in 1986, Zoya was the first line to remove toxic ingredients such as toluene, camphor, formaldehyde, and DBP from its formulations.
Where to buy it: Zoya (www.zoya.com)

Baby-Smart Products

Wipes
BabyGanics Thick N' Kleen Wipes
Why we love it: Seriously, these are the thickest wipes we've ever used! The worry-free formula is awesome at cleaning tushies, chins, hands, and everything in between. We also love the packaging. The lidded soft pack makes transporting them in our diaper bags super-easy.
Where to buy it: BabyGanics (www.babyganics.com)

Earth's Best TenderCare Chlorine-Free Wipes
Why we love it: We're big fans of the entire Earth's Best family of products. (The Earth's Best organic baby food is stellar.) Its thick wipes actually stay moist after the package has been opened. The natural vitamin E lotion is great at soothing our kids' tushies.
Where to buy it: Earth's Best (www.earthsbest.com)

Natracare Organic Cotton Baby Wipes
Why we love it: Made with 100 percent certified organic cotton, these dermatologist-tested wipes might be the softest we've ever encountered. Naturally gorgeously scented, thanks to an infusion of apricot, linden, and chamomile essential oils, these wipes are ones we couldn't stop sniffing.
    Where to buy it: Drugstore.com (www.drugstore.com)

Pampers Sensitive Wipes
Why we love it: We were thrilled to find a mild, baby-safe wipe from a brand that's been around for ages. These were the first wipes Melissa used on her first son when he was born. Pampers now offers Sensitive ThickCare wipes, which are awesome for cleaning up the yuckier diaper messes.
    Where to buy it: Diapers.com (www.diapers.com)

Diaper Cream

BabyGanics Hiney Helper Diaper Cream
Why we love it: A no-nonsense, xenoestrogen-free diaper cream that really gets the job done. After using it on our little ones' irritated bums, we saw a marked improvement by the next day!
    Where to buy it: BabyGanics (www.babyganics.com)

Lavanila: The Healthy Baby Bottom
Why we love it: We are thrilled that Lavanila created a baby care line. This synthetic-free diaper cream appeals to all our senses. It's safe for baby, the soothing formula feels luxurious, and it's quite a looker. We care a lot more about the ingredients than about the packaging, but this lovely diaper cream comes housed in a chic little tube.
    Where to buy: Lavanila (www.lavanila.com)

Method Baby Squeaky Green Diaper Cream
Why we love it: We count on Method for almost all of our household needs. Its super-savvy, eco-friendly products are some of the best around. We love Method's diaper cream, which comes in a smart pump dispenser and coats the tushie without any greasy residue. Moms who use cloth diapers love this cream because it doesn't leave a stain.
    Where to buy it: Method (www.methodhome.com)

Shampoo/Body Wash

BabyGanics Foamin' Fun Newborn Bodywash and
Shampoo Fragrance Free
Why we love it: Not only is this playful body wash made with smart ingredients, but it's also really fun to use. Once you pull open the applicator cap and squeeze the bottle, the foaming fun begins.
    Where to buy it: BabyGanics (www.babyganics.com)

Babo Botanicals Oatmilk Calendula Moisturizing Baby
Shampoo and Wash
Why we love it: Made with a soothing blend of chamomile, watercress, and calendula, plus oatmilk to comfort dry, chapped skin, this shampoo-and-body-wash combo has quickly become one of our favorites. Our babies' skin always feels deliciously soft after washing them with this.
    Where to buy it: Babo Botanicals (www.babobotanicals.com)

Belli Baby Calm Me Hair and Body Wash
Why we love it: This gentle cleanser handles baby's skin with kid gloves. The milk-and-honey essence is exactly the delicious scent you want to smell when you kiss the top of your little one's head.
    Where to buy it: Belli (www.belliskincare.com)

Exederm Baby Eczema Wash

Why we love it: We don't like to take any chances with our babies' skin, which is why it's so important to us to use only the mildest ingredients. Exederm, which is recognized by the National Eczema Association, created this nondrying, soap-free wash for children with the most sensitive skin.

Where to buy it: Exederm (www.exederm.com)

Taslie Head to Toe Body Wash

Why we love it: Taslie founder Tami Main puts her heart into the making of all her baby-friendly products, and this wash is no exception. The amazing nonsynthetic scent comes courtesy of an organic blend of mandarin and vanilla essential oils. We especially love the recyclable turtle pump bottle, which actually makes hand washing fun for our older sons.

Where to buy it: Taslie Skin Care (www.taslie.com)

Sunblock: Kids

Babo Botanicals Clear Zinc Sport Stick SPF 30 Sun and Wind Protection

Why we love it: It's pretty darn hard to find an invisible, synthetic-free sun protector that's not made with nanoparticles, but the mom-preneur behind Babo Botanicals was able to produce one, and now we're obsessed with it! This portable stick is a diaper bag staple if there ever was one. It's the perfect protector for the face, lips, nose, and ears. Shea butter and beeswax help soothe chapped skin during both summer and winter. And the best part is that our kids actually love applying it themselves.

Where to buy it: Babo Botanicals (www.babobotanicals.com)

Episencial Sunny Sunscreen SPF 35
Why we love it: You'd never know from the smooth, milky texture that this sunblock is made from zinc and titanium minerals. Besides blocking UVA/UVB rays, it moisturizes the skin thanks to baby-smart sesame and avocado oils.
Where to buy it: Episencial (www.episencial.com)

Lavanila Healthy Baby Block SPF 40
Why we love it: This elegantly formulated, vitamin-rich sunscreen went quickly in our households, probably because we were using it on the whole family. The pediatrician-approved formula is so clean that Melissa even used it on her newborn.
Where to buy it: Lavanila (www.lavanila.com)

Dr. Robin for Kids All-Natural Chemical-Free Sunscreen SPF 30+
Why we love it: If there's someone who knows about safe sunscreen for kids, it's pediatric dermatologist Dr. Robin Schaffran. Her water-resistant formula is made without parabens, fragrance, or synthetic chemicals of any sort. We feel safe letting our kids run around all day at the beach if they're covered with Dr. Robin.
Where to buy it: Dr. Robin for Kids (www.drrobin.md)

Baby Lotion

Babo Botanicals Oatmilk Calendula Moisturizing Body Lotion
Why we love it: This is a fabulous scalp treatment for babies! It's made with colloidal oatmeal, an amazing baby-smart ingredient that soothes and comforts dry skin. The calendula and shea butter are great for relieving cradle cap.
Where to buy: Babo Botanicals (www.babobotanicals.com)

Belli Baby Nourish Me Enriched Body Lotion

Why we love it: The ultimate soothing moisturizer for baby's face and body. We use it nightly after bath time to give our boys a light massage—it puts them right into a dreamlike trance!

Where to buy it: Belli (www.belliskincare.com)

Exederm Hydrating Baby Lotion

Why we love it: The folks at Exederm don't take any chances with their ingredients. This super-mild lotion, which is formulated without any harsh chemicals, dyes, or fragrance, is a must for babies with ultra-sensitive skin or for anyone who suffers from eczema. We've been using it on our own dry patches, and it's been working wonders!

Where to buy it: Exederm (www.exederm.com)

Taslie Moisturizing Lotion

Why we love it: This is quite possibly the fastest-absorbing body lotion we've tried. It literally melts into the skin without leaving a trace of greasiness behind. Plus, the mandarin and vanilla essential oils smell heavenly!

Where to buy it: Taslie Skin Care (www.taslie.com)

Acknowledgments

Annette

With heartfelt thanks to my sons Jackson and Cody, who inspired me to create Belli, and to my husband Jason, who made it all possible.

A debt of gratitude to Dayna for standing by me through thick and thin and to Melissa for her patience and her passion.

My deepest appreciation goes to my mother, who supported me, believed in me, and also introduced me at a young age to pink spongy curlers and Avon's pin pals solid perfumes. This resulted in my lifetime love and curiosity for all things designed to help women be a more beautiful version of themselves.

Melissa

Thank you to my coauthor, Annette. You inspired me to make improvements—big and small—to my life before my first baby, and you've literally been there with me every step along the way to listen and share the woes of motherhood. Your generosity is almost as limitless as your enthusiasm and brilliance. I couldn't ask for a better work partner and friend. You made this book a true labor of love.

Thanks to Dr. Jason Rubin, whose pioneering research is at the heart of this book. It's been a great pleasure to work with you. Your wonderful ideas, high standards, and exemplary ethics make this book a true force.

A heartfelt thank-you to my mentor and friend, the late Charla Krupp. She was an inspiration, a talented writer, and a guiding light who always pushed me to be a better journalist.

To my mom and dad—without you, this book would not have been possible. Thank you for your unyielding support and love. I look forward to enduring future moments of embarrassment when you tell the waitress that your daughter is an author.

To my brother and dermatologist Eric—thank you for helping me tackle my own skin issues during pregnancy and beyond. I will be counting on you to keep me looking young no matter how old my kids get.

A huge kiss to my biggest cheerleader, my husband Mitch. Thank you for giving me two beautiful, loving, and tireless little boys, and thank you for taking care of those boys when I needed the house to myself to work on the book. You have been nothing but supportive and terrific throughout the whole book-writing process. Your suggestions and guidance helped to make this book my most crowning achievement—not to be outdone by our family.

To Jonah and Ilan, my two little munchkins. This book is dedicated to you. They say motherhood is the toughest job you'll ever love—and they're right. I'm lucky to have two perfect beings who tear at my heartstrings and bring indescribable joy—along with fleeting moments of hair-pulling frustration—to every single day.

Melissa and Annette

We'd like to thank Eileen Cope for her support, enthusiasm, and guidance. She was excited about the idea from the start and has been there for us every step of the way.

Thanks also to the team at Da Capo Lifelong Books. Thanks to Katie McHugh for her brilliant edits and for pushing us to make the book the very best that it could be. A big thank-you to Annie Lenth, Cynthia Buck, and Kevin Hanover.

Thanks to all of our amazing contributors. We wouldn't have been able to write this book without your incredible insights, funny anecdotes, and genius tips. You have inspired us in so many ways!

Notes

Introduction

1. J. Houlihan et al., "Body Burden—The Pollution in Newborns," Environmental Working Group, July 14, 2005. This paper analyzes tests of ten umbilical cord blood samples that were conducted by AXYS Analytical Services (Sydney, British Columbia) and Flett Research Ltd. (Winnipeg, Manitoba).

Chapter 1: Healthy Beauty for a Healthy Pregnancy

1. US Food and Drug Administration, "FDA Authority over Cosmetics," March 3, 2005, http://www.fda.gov/Cosmetics/GuidanceCompliance RegulatoryInformation/ucm074162.htm.

2. Cosmetic Ingredient Review, http://www.cir-safety.org.

3. The Campaign for Safe Cosmetics, "FDA Regulations," http://safe cosmetics.org/section.php?id=75.

4. T. H. Shephard and R. J. Lemire, *Catalog of Teratogenic Agents*, 11th ed. (Baltimore: Johns Hopkins University Press, 2004); G. G. Briggs, R. K. Freeman, and S. J. Yaffe, *Drugs in Pregnancy and Lactation: A Reference Guide to Fetal and Neonatal Risks*, 8th ed. (Philadelphia: Lippincott Williams & Wilkins, 2008); J. Schardein, *Chemically Induced Birth Defects*, 3rd ed. (New York: Marcel Dekker, 2000).

5. US Food and Drug Administration, "Cosmetics: Product and Ingredient Safety," http://www.fda.gov/Cosmetics/ProductandIngredientSafety/ProductInformation/ucm203078.htm.

Chapter 2: Ingredient Watch

1. FD&C Act, sec. 201.

2. K. S. Kang et al., "Decreased Sperm Number and Motility Activity on the F1 Offspring Maternally Exposed to Butyl p-Hydroxybenzoic Acid (Butylparaben)," *Journal of Veterinary Medical Science* 64, no. 3 (March 2002): 22–35.

3. S. Oishi, "Effects of Propyl Paraben on the Male Reproductive System," *Food and Chemical Toxicology* 40, no. 12 (December 2002): 1807–1813.

4. S. Oishi, "Effects of Butyl Paraben on the Male Reproductive System in Mice," *Archives of Toxicology* 76, no. 7 (July 2002): 423–429.

5. J. R. Byford et al., "Oestrogenic Activity of Parabens in MCF7 Human Breast Cancer Cells," *Journal of Steroid Biochemistry and Molecular Biology* 80, no. 1 (January 2002): 49–60.

6. E. J. Routledge, J. Parker, J. Odum, et al., "Some Alkyl Hydroxy Benzoate Preservatives (Parabens) Are Estrogenic," *Toxicology and Applied Pharmacology* 153, no. 1 (November 1998): 12–19.

7. I. Colón, D. Caro, C. J. Bourdony, and O. Rosario, "Identification of Phthalate Esters in the Serum of Young Puerto Rican Girls with Premature Breast Development," *Environmental Health Perspectives* 108, no. 9 (September 2000): 895–900.

8. R. Hauser, J. D. Meeker, S. Duty, et al., "Altered Semen Quality in Relation to Urinary Concentrations of Phthalate Monoester and Oxidative Metabolites," *Epidemiology* 17, no. 6 (November 2006): 682–691.

9. G. Delbes, C. Levacher, and R. Habert, "Estrogen Effects on Fetal and Neonatal Testicular Development," *Reproduction* 132, no. 4 (October 2006): 527–538.

10. S. H. Swan et al., "Decrease in Anogenital Distance Among Male Infants with Prenatal Phthalate Exposure," *Environmental Health Perspectives* 113, no. 8 (August 2005), doi:10.1289/ehp.8100.

11. S. Y. Euling, S. G. Selevan, O. H. Pescovitz, and N. E. Skakkebaek, "Role of Environmental Factors in the Timing of Puberty," *Pediatrics* 121 (supplement, February 2008): S167–S171.

12. T. J. Gray and K. R. Butterworth, "Testicular Atrophy Produced by Phthalate Esters," *Archives of Toxicology Supplement* 4 (1980): 452–455.

13. A. El-Mubarak and D. Huisingh, "Environmental Xenoestrogens: Short-Term Exposure of Low Doses of Lindane, Dieldrin, Dibutyl Phthalate, and Diethylhexyl Phthalate Increases Uterine Weight in Young Female Mice," *Analytical Sciences* 17 (ICAS2001): i261.

14. S. Sathyanarayana et al., "Baby Care Products: Possible Sources of Infant Phthalate Exposure," *Pediatrics* 121, no. 2 (February 2008): e260–e268.

15. EWG's Skin Deep Cosmetics Database, http://www.ewg.org /skindeep/ingredient/726331/1,4-DIOXANE/#.

16. M. Schlumpf et al., "In Vitro and In Vivo Estrogenicity of UV Screens," *Environmental Health Perspectives* 109, no. 3 (March 2001): 239–244.

17. H. Matsumoto, S. Adachi, and Y. Suzuki, "Estrogenic Activity of Ultraviolet Absorbers and the Related Compounds," *Yakugaku Zasshi* 125, no. 8 (August 2005): 643–652.

18. P. Y. Kunz and K. Fent, "Multiple Hormonal Activities of UV Filters and Comparison of In Vivo and In Vitro Estrogenic Activity of Ethyl-4-Aminobenzoate in Fish," *Aquatic Toxicology* 79, no. 4 (October 12, 2006): 305–324, published online June 30, 2006.

19. E. Cekanova, K. S. Larsson, E. Orck, and G. Aberg, "Interactions Between Salicylic Acid and Pyridyl-3-Methanol: Anti-inflammatory and Teratogenic Effects," *Acta Pharmacology and Toxicology* 35, no. 2 (1974): 107–118.

20. D. Overman and J. White, "Comparative Teratogenic Effects of Methyl Salicylate Applied Orally or Topically to Hamsters," *Teratology* 28, no. 3 (December 1983): 421–426.

21. D. R. Newall and J. R. Edwards, "The Effect of Vitamin A on Fusion of Mouse Palates. I. Retinyl Palmitate and Retinoic Acid In Vivo," *Teratology* 23, no. 1 (1981): 115–124.

22. A. H. Piersma, W. Bode, A. Verhoef, and M. Olling, "Teratogenicity of a Single Oral Dose of Retinyl Palmitate in the Rat, and the Role of Dietary Vitamin A Status," *Pharmacology and Toxicology* 79, no. 3 (1996): 131–135.

23. Propylene glycol (REPROTEXT® document), in REPROTEXT® database, ed. G. Heitland and K. M. Hurlbut (Greenwood Village, CO: MICROMEDEX, edition expired June 2003).

24. S. Song et al., "Combined Repeated Dose and Reproductive/ Developmental Toxicities of Benzoyl Peroxide," *Journal of Toxicology and Public Health: An Official Journal of the Korean Society of Toxicology* 19, no. 2 (2003): 123–131.

25. A. R. Gasset and T. Akaboshi, "Embryopathic Effect of Ophthalmic EDTA," *Investigative Ophthalmology and Visual Science* 16, no. 7 (1977): 652–654.

26. H. Swenerton and L. S. Hurley, "Teratogenic Effects of a Chelating Agent and Their Prevention by Zinc," *Science* 173, no. 991 (1971): 62–64.

27. D. Nath, N. Sethi, R. K. Singh, and A. K. Jain, "Commonly Used Indian Abortifacient Plants with Special Reference to Their Teratologic Effects in Rats," *Journal of Ethnopharmacology* 36 (1992): 147–154.

28. M. K. Nusier, H. N. Bataineh, and H. M. Daradkah, "Adverse Effects of Rosemary (*Rosmarinus officinalis* OL) on Reproductive Function in Adult Male Rats," *Experimental Biology and Medicine* (Maywood) 232, no. 6 (2007): 809–813.

29. W. D. Brown, A. R. Johnson, and M. W. O'Halloran, "The Effect of the Level of Dietary Fat on the Toxicity of Phenolic Antioxidants," *Australian Journal of Experimental Biology and Medical Science* 37 (1959): 533–547.

30. J. D. Stokes and C. L. Scudder, "The Effect of Butylated Hydroxyanisole and Butylated Hydroxytoluene on Behavioral Development of Mice," *Developmental Psychobiology* 7, no. 4 (1974): 343–350.

31. G. L. Kennedy Jr., M. L. Keplinger, J. C. Calandra, and E. J. Hobbs, "Reproductive, Teratologic, and Mutagenic Studies with Some Polydimethylsiloxanes," *Journal of Toxicology and Environmental Health* 1, no. 6 (1976): 909–920.

32. K. Oba and R. Takei, "Carcinogenic, Mutagenic/Genetic Toxicity, and Teratogenic Properties," in *Anionic Surfactants: Biochemistry, Toxicol-*

ogy, *Dermatology*, 2nd ed., ed. C. Gloxhuber and K. Kuenstler (New York: Marcel Dekker, 1992), pp. 331–409.

33. "Final Report on the Safety Assessment of Sodium Lauryl Sulfate and Ammonium Lauryl Sulfate," *Journal of the American College of Toxicology* 2, no. 7 (1983): 127–181.

34. U. Kocher-Becker, W. Kocher, and H. Ockenfels, "Thalidomide-like Malformations Caused by Tween Surfactant in Mice," *Zeitschrift für Naturforsche* 36, nos. 9–10 (1981): 904–906.

35. J. M. Wilkinson, "Effect of Ginger Tea on the Fetal Development of Sprague-Dawley Rats," *Reproductive Toxicology* 14, no. 6 (2000): 507–512.

36. S. M. Munley, G. L. Kennedy, and M. E. Hurtt, "Developmental Toxicity Study of Glycolic Acid in Rats," *Drug and Chemical Toxicology* 22, no. 4 (1999): 569–582.

37. D. K. Gulati, R. Mounce, R. E. Chapin, and J. Heindel, "Final Report on the Reproductive Toxicity of 2-Hydroxy-4-Methoxybenzophenone (CAS no. 131-57-7) in CD-1-Swiss Mice," NTIS (National Technical Information Service) report PB91-158477 (1990).

38. Kang et al., "Decreased Sperm Number and Motility Activity on the F1 Offspring Maternally Exposed to Butyl p-Hydroxybenzoic Acid (Butylparaben)."

39. S. K. Garg and G. P. Garg, "Antifertility Screening of Plants. Part VII. Effect of Five Indigenous Plants on Early Pregnancy in Albino Rats," *Indian Journal of Medical Research* 59 (1970): 302–306.

40. J. D. Singh, "Palm Oil Induced Congenital Anomalies in Rats," *Congenital Anomalies* (1980): 139–142.

Chapter 3: Mom-Smart Facial Care

1. S. Trauer et al., "Permeation of Topically Applied Caffeine Through Human Skin: A Comparison of In Vivo and In Vitro Data," *Journal of Clinical Pharmacology* 68, no. 2 (August 2009): 181–186, http://www.ncbi.nlm.nih.gov/pmc/articles/PMC2767280/.

2. X. Weng, R. Odouli, and D. K. Li, "Maternal Caffeine Consumption During Pregnancy and the Risk of Miscarriage: A Prospective Cohort

Study," *American Journal of Obstetrics and Gynecology* 198, no. 3 (March 2008): 279.e1–8, http://www.ncbi.nlm.nih.gov/pubmed/18221932.

3. Environmental Working Group, "Impurities of Concern in Personal Care Products," 2006.

4. B. J. Shaw and R. D. Handy, "Physiological Effects of Nanoparticles on Fish: A Comparison of Nanometals Versus Metal Ions," *Environment International* 37, no. 6 (August 2011): 1083–1097, http://www.ncbi.nlm.nih.gov/pubmed/21474182.

Chapter 4: Mom-Smart Body and Hair Care

1. S. Offenbacher et al., "Periodontitis: A Potential Risk Factor for Spontaneous Preterm Birth," *Compendium of Continuing Education in Dentistry* 19, no. 1 (1999): 32–39.

2. E. Lerner, "Penn Research Shows Mouthwash Routine May Cut Risk of Preterm Birth," *Penn News*, October 27, 2011, http://www.upenn.edu/pennnews/news/penn-research-shows-mouthwash-routine-may-cut-risk-preterm-birth.

3. X. Liu, J. E. Grice, and J. Lademann, "Hair Follicles Contribute Significantly to Penetration Through Human Skin Only at Times Soon After Application as a Solvent Deposited Solid in Man," *British Journal of Clinical Pharmacology* 72, no. 5 (November 2011): 768–774.

4. K. He, J. Huang, C. F. Lagenaur, and E. Aizenman, "Methylisothiazolinone, a Neurotoxic Biocide, Disrupts the Association of SRC Family Tyrosine Kinases with Focal Adhesion Kinase in Developing Cortical Neurons," *Journal of Pharmacology and Experimental Therapeutics* 317 (2006): 1320–1329.

5. G. Ormond et al., "Endocrine Disruptors in the Workplace, Hair Spray, Folate Supplementation, and Risk of Hypospadias: Case-Control Study," *Environmental Health Perspectives* 117, no. 2 (February 2009): 303–307, published online November 20, 2008.

6. US Food and Drug Administration, "Triclosan: What Consumers Should Know," April 8, 2010, http://www.fda.gov/forconsumers/consumerupdates/ucm205999.htm.

7. UC Davis, "Antibacterial Chemical Disrupts Hormone Activities," December 7, 2007, http://www.news.ucdavis.edu/search/news_detail .lasso?id=8456.

8. K. Koecher and D. Krenke, "A Comparative Study of the Immediate Effects of a Triclosan Antibacterial, Chloroxylenol Antibacterial, and Lotion Soap," 2000, murphylibrary.uwlax.edu/digital/jur/2000/koecher-krenke .pdf.

9. A. C. Steinemann et al., "Fragranced Consumer Products: Chemicals Emitted, Ingredients Unlisted," *Environmental Impact Assessment Review* (2010), doi:10.1016/j.eiar.2010.08.002.

10. T. Komori et al., "Effects of Citrus Fragrance on Immune Function and Depressive States," *Neuroimmunomodulation* 2, no. 3 (May–June 1995): 174–180.

11. Candida Research and Information Foundation, Perfume Survey, Winter 1989–90, compiled by comparing a list of 120 fragrance chemicals from the EPA obtained through the Freedom of Information Act and California's Prop 65 List of Chemicals.

12. H. Osman, A. Usta, N. Rubiez, et al., "Cocoa Butter Lotion for Prevention of *Striae gravidarum*: A Double-Blind, Randomized, and Placebo-Controlled Trial," *British Journal of Gynecology* 115 (2008): 1138–1142.

13. J. Mallol, M. Belda, D. Costa, et al., "Prophylaxis of *Striae gravidarum* with a Topical Formulation: A Double-Blind Trial," *International Journal of Cosmetic Science* 13 (1991): 51–57.

14. Darutoside and registril research studies were conducted by Phybotex Labs, Sederma Group, France, 1997. Data on file.

15. "Breastfeeding and Maternal and Infant Health Outcomes in Developed Countries," Evidence Report/Technology Assessment 153, prepared for US Department of Health and Human Services, Agency for Healthcare Research and Quality by Tufts–New England Medical Center Evidence-Based Practice Center, Boston, April 2007.

16. J. H. Clark and W. G. Wilson, "A 16-Day-Old Breast-Fed Infant with Metabolic Acidosis Caused by Salicylate," *Clinical Pediatrics* 20 (1981): 53–54.

17. A. Terragna and L. Spirito, "Porpora Trombocitopenica in Lattante Dopo Somministrazione di Acido Acetilsalicilico alla Nutrice" ("Thrombocytopenic Purpura in an Infant After Administration of Acetylsalicylic Acid to the Wet-Nurse"), *Minerva Pediatrica* 19 (1967): 613–616.

18. J. D. Harley and H. Robin, "'Late' Neonatal Jaundice in Infants with Glucose-6-Phosphate Dehydrogenase-Deficient Erythrocytes," *Australasian Annals of Medicine* 11 (1962): 148–155.

19. R. Knutti, H. Rothweiler, and C. H. Schlatter, "Effect of Pregnancy on the Pharmacokinetics of Caffeine," *European Journal of Clinical Pharmacology* 21 (1981): 121–126.

20. D. N. Bailey, R. T. Welbert, and A. Naylor, "A Study of Salicylate and Caffeine Excretion in the Breast Milk of Two Nursing Mothers," *Journal of Analytical Toxicology* 6 (1982): 64–68.

21. M. I. Clement, "Caffeine and Babies," *British Medical Journal* 298 (1989): 1461.

22. J. Rustin, "Caffeine and Babies" (letter), *British Medical Journal* 299 (1989): 121.

23. L. M. Munoz, B. Lonnerdal, C. L. Keen, and K. G. Dewey, "Coffee Consumption as a Factor in Iron Deficiency Anemia Among Pregnant Women and Their Infants in Costa Rica," *American Journal of Clinical Nutrition* 48 (1988): 645–651.

Chapter 5: Mom-Smart Makeup

1. D. McCann, A. Barrett, A. Cooper, et al., "Food Additives and Hyperactive Behaviour in Three-Year-Old and Eight- to Nine-Year-Old Children in the Community: A Randomised, Double-Blinded, Placebo-Controlled Trial," *Lancet* 370 (2007): 1560–1567.

2. G. Schlüter, "Embryotoxic Action of Carmine in Mice," *Z Anat Entwicklungsgesch* 131, no. 3 (1970): 228–235.

3. World Health Organization, "Mercury in Skin Lightening Products," September 2011, http://www.who.int/ipcs/assessment/public_health /mercury_flyer.pdf.

4. N. L. Etcoff, S. Stock, L. E. Haley, S. A. Vickery, and D. M. House, "Cosmetics as a Feature of the Extended Human Phenotype: Modulation of the Perception of Biologically Important Facial Signals," *PLoS ONE* 6, no. 10 (2011): e25656.

Chapter 6: Staying Smart at the Salon and Spa: Nails, Hair, Massage, and More

1. US Food and Drug Administration, "Summary of Regulatory Requirements for Labeling of Cosmetics Marketed in the United States," October 1991, updated June 2009 and April 2011, http://www.fda.gov/Cosmetics/CosmeticLabelingLabelClaims/CosmeticLabelingManual/ucm126438.htm.

2. M. Tang, Y. Xie, Y. Yi, and W. Wang, "Effects of Formaldehyde on Germ Cells of Male Mice," *Wei Sheng Yan Jiu* 32, no. 6 (November 2003): 544–548, http://www.ncbi.nlm.nih.gov/pubmed/14963899; E. M. John et al., "Spontaneous Abortions Among Cosmetologists," *Epidemiology* 5, no. 2 (1994): 147–155.

Chapter 7: Baby-Smart Skin Care

1. For more information on efforts to persuade Congress to reform the law, watch the "Take Out Toxics" video at the Natural Resources Defense Council website (www.takeouttoxics.org).

Meet the Experts

We turned to these top experts in the fields of beauty, skin care, and medicine in the writing of this book. Through extensive interviews and many emails, they answered all of our questions and armed us with much of the vital information you'll glean from each chapter.

Dr. Jason Rubin

Jason Rubin, MD, is the founding physician of Belli Skin Care. Working together with a team of other experts (obstetrician, dermatologist, and teratologist), he guided Belli's chemists in the creation of each unique product. He also wrote a series of educational articles that teach women about the skin care changes of pregnancy and motherhood and the best care and cleansing routines for their babies. Dr. Rubin received his medical degree from St. Louis University School of Medicine in 1997. He is now a board-certified family practitioner with broad experience in obstetrics, pediatrics, dermatology, and emergency medicine. He is an attending physician at Snoqualmie Valley Hospital in Washington State. Dr. Jason Rubin and Annette Rubin are the parents of two beautiful boys.

Penelope Jagessar Chaffer

When filmmaker Penelope Jagessar Chaffer discovered that she might be exposing her baby to life-threatening diseases and developmental disorders, she knew she had to share that information with the world. She sold her house to fund her documentary *Toxic Baby*, which follows her search for the truth about what all of the thousands of chemicals manufactured today might be doing to our children. During the making of the film, she traveled around the world for six years to interview scientists and doctors in an effort to establish that the effects of chemicals in the environment on our children are indeed a real issue. Penelope has been nominated for a BAFTA (the British Academy Award) and has received many other awards and accolades, including Healthy Child, Healthy World's 2010 "Mom on a Mission" award. She lives in New York City with her husband and two children.

Eva Scrivo

Eva Scrivo is the author of *Eva Scrivo on Beauty: The Tools, Techniques, and Insider Knowledge Every Woman Needs to Be Her Most Beautiful, Confident Self* (Atria Books, 2011). Additionally, she is a renowned hair and makeup artist, television and radio personality, and entrepreneur with an eponymous salon in New York City. Eva is a rare hands-on expert in haircutting, coloring, and makeup and has keen knowledge of skin care, nutrition, wellness, and fashion. Through her experience, range of expertise, charisma, and penchant for teaching, she has come to be regarded as one of the country's premier beauty experts. Uniquely qualified to share information on all aspects of beauty, Eva has served as the resident expert on NBC's *Martha* and appeared on shows such as CBS *Early Show, Good Morning America, Good Day New York, Greta Van Susteren,* and Lifetime's *The Balancing Act.* For six years she hosted a weekly one-hour talk show, *Beauty Talk,* on Sirius/XM Radio. Her work has been featured in magazines like *Vogue* and *Marie Claire,* and she has been profiled in *Vanity Fair, Allure,* and *Gotham,* among others. Especially known for the "makeover," Eva sees women from across the country at her salon. She is also a L'Oréal Professionnel Celebrity Stylist and Colorist and an elite-level educator at the L'Oréal academies.

Dr. Macrene Alexiades-Armenakas

Macrene Alexiades-Armenakas, MD, PhD, is one of the most sought-after dermatologists in the world. She received her three degrees from

Harvard University: a BA and a PhD in genetics from Harvard University and an MD from Harvard Medical School. She was a Fulbright Scholar with a research award year in Europe. She is a fellow of the American Academy of Dermatology and the American Society for Laser Medicine and Surgery. She is an assistant clinical professor at Yale University School of Medicine and an attending physician at Lenox Hill Hospital, Yale–New Haven Hospital, and Yale–West Haven VA Hospital. Dr. Alexiades-Armenakas founded and directs her dermatology, laser surgery, and research center in Manhattan and a lab-based skin care research company called NY Derm LLC. She's often featured in *Vogue, Elle, Allure,* and *InStyle.* She has also served as dermatologist and skin care expert for L'Oréal, Paris, with which she developed an acne skin care line. Dr. Alexiades-Armenakas, a mother of two, lives in New York City with her family.

Dr. Robin Schaffran

Robin Schaffran, MD, is a board-certified dermatologist who has been treating parents and children in her Beverly Hills private practice for over ten years. She is an attending staff physician at Cedars-Sinai Medical Center, and over the years she has developed an expertise in caring for children's skin. When she realized that there were very few products she felt comfortable recommending to her patients, she developed a line of children's skin care called Dr. Robin for Kids. She has lectured extensively on the subject of skin cancer prevention and has been quoted in publications like the *Los Angeles Times* and *US News & World Report.* Dr. Schaffran was born and raised in Toronto and attended McGill University in Montreal. She went on to the University of Toronto Medical School, where she graduated as a member of the Alpha-Omega-Alpha Honors Medical Society. After completing her internal medicine internship at Beth Israel Hospital of Harvard Medical School, she finished her residency dermatology training at the Oregon Health Sciences University in Portland. Dr. Schaffran lives in Los Angeles with her husband and children. Whenever possible, she relaxes in the shade under an umbrella or tree.

Dr. Janine Polifka

Dr. Janine Polifka has been the codirector of CARE Northwest, a teratogen information service located at the University of Washington. She also manages the TERIS database, which provides up-to-date, authoritative information regarding the effects of drugs and chemicals on the developing embryo. Dr. Polifka is the cochair of the research committee of the Organization of Teratology Information Specialists, a national organization that oversees fifteen teratology information services throughout the United States and Canada. She previously served on the public affairs committee of the Teratology Society.

Nonie Crème

Founding creative director of Butter London, Nonie Crème is the transatlantic brand's ambassador. With experience from product design and development to packaging design and press relations, she leads all creative efforts and keeps the messaging and artistry unequivocally British. Since the company's conception, Nonie has been at the helm of all formulation and design endeavors, using imaginative techniques, bold graphics, and audacious cheeky humor to make the Butter London line a modern cult classic. Her innovations in color and merchandise have helped shape the industry. Nonie holds a BA in art history and fine arts from Scripps University in California and has a three-year-old daughter, Paloma, who loves nail polish almost as much as her mum does!

Dr. Jonathan Levine

When it comes to cosmetic dentistry, Dr. Levine is our go-to guy. As a renowned aesthetic dentist and prosthodontist in practice for nearly thirty years, Dr. Levine takes a comprehensive approach to dental health at the intersection of beauty and function. He's a visionary product inventor (for instance, he's the genius behind Glo Science), a clinical researcher, and a published author. He holds five patents and has twelve patents pending in oral care. Dr. Levine is an associate professor at the New York University School of Dentistry and the program director of the Advanced Aesthetics Program in Dentistry at the NYU School of Continuing Education. Dr. Levine has appeared on several national television networks and shows, including CNN, *Good Morning America, The Dr. Oz Show* (as an oral health and smile expert), and *The View.* As an authoritative source on smile health and beauty, he is frequently quoted in top national print publications, including *InStyle, Marie Claire, Men's Health, People Stylewatch, Self,* the *New York Times,* and *USA Today.* Dr. Levine is the author of *Smile Design and the Language of Esthetics,* as well as two other published books, and dad to two college-age sons.

Dr. David Abel

Dr. David Abel is a perinatologist at the Deaconess Medical Center in Spokane, Washington. He graduated Phi Beta Kappa from Tufts University. Dr. Abel earned his medical degree from Syracuse University and did his ob-gyn residency at Maine Medical Center in Portland. He completed a fellowship in maternal-fetal medicine at Duke University and was a chief ob-gyn at Copley Hospital in Vermont. Dr. Abel lives with his wife and son in Portland, Oregon.

Kate Somerville

Kate Somerville's name is synonymous with perfect skin. Her Los Angeles medi-spa, Kate Somerville Skin Health Experts, is a hugely successful skin clinic in Los Angeles that draws some of Hollywood's most famous faces. By partnering with top dermatologists and cosmetic surgeons and promoting the integration of skin care and medicine, she pioneered the field of paramedical aesthetics and helped lay the foundation for the medi-spa industry. Kate's multidimensional strategy for achieving healthy skin has made her one of the most trusted names in skin care today. A mom herself, Kate is personally responsible for the gorgeous complexions of other hot mamas, including Jessica Alba and Debra Messing.

Janet Markovits

Janet Markovits has been a New York State licensed massage therapist since 1997. A graduate of the Swedish Institute of Massage, Janet is nationally certified in therapeutic massage and bodywork and is a member of the American Massage Therapy Association. She has studied numerous modalities, including MotherMassage® with Elaine Stillerman, Mayan abdominal massage with Rosita Arvigo, cranio-sacral and lymphatic drainage with the Upledger Institute, and sports massage with James Hackett. Her practice, Maternal Massage and More, has been featured on the *Channel 11 Morning News* and on *ABC News*. Janet is an expert in the massage field and has been featured in numerous magazines. She is also the host of *From Here to Maternity* on the VoiceAmerica Health and Wellness Channel. Janet continues to educate herself and her clients on the latest techniques and research. She is founder of The Pregnant New Yorker, which provides alternative, fun health events in New York City and Brooklyn.

Kevin Schwartz and Keith Garber

Kevin Schwartz and Keith Garber are the founding fathers of BabyGanics. Kevin's vision of creating household solutions that are both earth-friendly and people-friendly began when he became increasingly aware of the alarming rates of childhood illness related to the chemicals used in our homes. He saw the opportunity to create a business that would encourage parent education while simultaneously having a positive impact on the lives of growing families everywhere. BabyGanics was born out of his passion and commitment to creating a range of safe, effective, and affordable products. Keith Garber is a passionate supporter of health, wellness, and sustainability. A seasoned entrepreneur, Keith's personal mission was also to help create a business venture that would have a positive impact on people's lives. He joined forces with Kevin with the goal of expanding the BabyGanics product assortment and building distribution to provide parents with solutions in numerous areas of their lives. With his steadfast commitment to spreading the BabyGanics vision, he has helped give consumers the opportunity to provide their families with safe, natural, and accessible solutions for creating healthier home environments.

Laura Geller

Early on, Laura Geller knew that her future would be in makeup. Her path took her from beauty school to Broadway, where she made up the theater industry's rising stars and soon became one of the industry's top makeup artists. Soon after, Laura's artistry also graced the on-air talent featured on television shows, including NBC's *Today Show* in New York and shows on CBS, CW, and HBO. Today Laura is mostly found in front of the camera through her many QVC appearances in the United States and internationally. She has taken QVC Europe by storm as the United Kingdom's fastest-selling makeup brand. Not only is Laura hands-on in all aspects of her namesake brand, but she also operates an Upper East Side studio, a must-visit destination for both her New York City clientele and fans from around the world who stop by to catch a glimpse of the glamorous place that started it all. Laura lives in New York City, where she's constantly balancing her life as a busy mom, makeup artist, and beauty entrepreneur. You'll see her on the soccer field cheering on her eleven-year-old son, sometimes in a full face of makeup.

Josie Maran

Supermodel, actress, activist, and eco-entrepreneur Josie Maran grew up appreciating natural, unpretentious beauty in a bohemian Northern California household. This natural take on beauty and a fresh attitude later landed Josie some of the most coveted jobs in the modeling industry, and she appeared on the covers of countless beauty and fashion magazines. Traveling the world as a model, Josie always sought out the best natural beauty secrets and ingredients. She struck gold while on a shoot in the South of France. Josie says: "I noticed an older woman with beautiful skin. She looked forty, and she was probably closer to seventy! I had to have her secret. She told me about argan oil, known as 'Moroccan Liquid Gold.' I've been hooked ever since! It's been my beauty secret for years!"

The birth of Josie's daughter, coupled with her own mom's natural take on beauty, inspired her to create Josie Maran Cosmetics. "Becoming a mother inspired me to take a look at my life and ask, 'What can I do for the world? How can I contribute?'" says Josie. Using the trade secrets she had amassed over her career, Josie created her own signature line of responsible, argan oil–based skin care and cosmetics. Josie embraces eco-friendly initiatives, formulates each of her products with superior ingredients, and takes great care to balance luxury with consciousness.

Lois Joy Johnson

Lois Joy Johnson is a top beauty editor, writer, author, and true product junkie. She was a founding editor and beauty and fashion director of *More* magazine and loves helping women deal with their beauty choices, issues, and dilemmas. She is the author of *The Makeup Wakeup: Revitalizing Your Look at Any Age* (Running Press), a beauty book geared for women entering their forties and beyond.

Maureen Kelly

A natural-born beauty junkie and entrepreneur at heart, Maureen Kelly became frustrated with what she witnessed on the market: unhealthy makeup sold in unglamorous black pots. So she set out to create Tarte, a line that proves glamour can be good for you. Launched in Manhattan-based department store Henri Bendel in September 2000, Tarte was immediately praised for its pure ingredients, powerful formulas, innovative packaging, impressive color range, chic portability, and cheeky names. At Tarte, everything Maureen creates is pure and performs with a purpose. She's committed to infusing wholesome ingredients—fruit and plant extracts, vitamins, minerals, essential oils, and other naturally derived ingredients—into all Tarte products. And when she says "pure" she also means that Tarte products are always formulated without parabens, phthalates, mineral oil, sodium lauryl sulfate, or synthetic fragrances. Maureen lives in New York with her husband and two sons.

Index

215